Pour the Water: Transformative Solutions for Equity & Justice in Special Education

Marcy Rachamim Jackson, MA

Pour the Water: Transformative Solutions for Equity & Justice in Special Education© 2024 Marcy Rachamim Jackson, MA

The Educational Leadership for Parents Model is protected by U.S. and International copyright law. © 2013 Marcy Jackson

All rights reserved. This book or parts thereof may not be reproduced in any form, stored in any retrieval system, or transmitted in any form by any means—electronic, mechanical, photocopy, recording, or otherwise—without prior written permission of the publisher, except as provided by United States of America copyright law or for the use of brief quotations in a book review.

Permission requests, inquiries for print copies, comments, or questions should be addressed to info@TheOlivez.com

Organizations may order print copies in bundles at a reduced cost.

Although the author and publisher have made every effort to ensure that the information in this book was correct at press time, the author and publisher do not assume and hereby disclaim any liability to any party for any loss, damage, or disruption caused by errors or omissions, whether such errors or omissions result from negligence, accident, or any other cause. Views expressed in this publication do not necessarily reflect the views of the publisher.

Printed in the United States of America

ISBN: 979-8-9896861-1-7
Marcy \Anderson-Jackson#OlivezEducationGrove

Contents

Introduction 5

Chapter 1 Perspectives on Education History 14

Chapter 2 Perspectives on Change in Systems, Practices, and People 37

Chapter 3 See the Pipeline: Decisions, Discipline, and Disparities 69

Chapter 4 Disconnect the School-to-Prison Pipeline: Align the School-to-Success Pathway 87

Chapter 5 Synchronize Health and Education: Solutions for Referral, Diet, and Stigma 111

Chapter 6 Educational Leadership for Parents and Professionals 137

Chapter 7 Education Equity Through Prioritization and Desire: Nine Passionate Priorities 159

Chapter 8 Universal Design and Accessibility: Inclusive Pedagogical Strategy 201

Chapter 9 Special Education Advocacy: Make Advocacy Accessible 219

Chapter 10 Transformed for Good: Conclusion with Recommendations 257

Appendix A Glossary of Acronyms and Related Terms 267

Appendix B Evidence-Based Interventions 271

Appendix C Disability Definitions from the Individuals with Disabilities Education Act (IDEA) Department of Education, Office of Special Education 275

Appendix D 2020 Initiative Charter for Special Education Excellence for Underserved Students (SEE US) . 281

Appendix E Interview with Advocate Rich Weinfeld 2022 .. 283

Appendix F Professional Development Graduate Course: Identifying and Removing Obstacles for Black Students with Special Needs..........289

Appendix G Interview with Professor Dr. Norell Edwards....295

References..........299

About the Author..........317

Introduction

Framework for Antiracist Policy and Practice

The United Nations Sustainable Development Goals (UNSDG) proclaims, "this is the time for change, for a profound systemic shift to a more sustainable economy, that works for both people and the planet." Education is the conduit towards developing professionals who will design and sustain this economy. By 2030, the UNSDG global priority for Quality Education (Goal 4) is to "ensure that all girls and boys complete free, equitable, and quality primary and secondary education leading to relevant and effective learning outcomes" (UNSDG). The United Nations International Children's Emergency Fund (UNICEF) demands that Goal 4 support the reduction of disparities and inequities in education, both in terms of access and quality. Specifically, UNICEF asks for "A continued commitment to improving access to pre-primary, primary, and secondary education for all, including for children from minority groups and those with disabilities" (UNSDG, 2023).

Inclusion or mainstreaming is supported nationally and globally as the way to help individuals with disabilities to thrive. According to UNESCO, "While 68% of countries have a definition of inclusive education, only 57% of those definitions cover multiple marginalized groups." *Pour the Water: Transformative Solutions for Equity & Justice in Special Education* directs attention toward the globally supported practice of inclusion through inclusive teaching, inclusive identification, and inclusive services for the most marginalized group of minorities, Black students with special needs.

Minority students with disabilities in the United States are largely educated in the public school system among typically developing peers.

Black students comprise most of the unidentified and underserved minority students with special needs within gifted, general, and special education settings. However, because of systemic racism, the subtlety of bias systematically stifles the processes and minority students with disabilities, gifts, and medical conditions are overlooked for services. Moreover, Black (along with Indigenous and Latinx) children are between six and nine times more likely than white children to live in areas of concentrated poverty (My Brother's Keeper Alliance, 2022).

However, all Black students with special needs (BSSNs) are not the same nor have the same group identity regarding ethnicity, racialized codes, culture, and special needs. Throughout your reading, you will find support for educators and practitioners to support individuality, uniqueness, and peculiarity. You will also see supported recommendations to disaggregate data to discern the issues and solutions, rather than continue with old methods.

For the reasons stated above, and more as presented in this book, Black students with special needs generally have poorer academic, functional, and behavioral outcomes. The lower rigor of academic programs, reduced services, and disparaging discipline practices across schools cause Black students with special needs to leave high school without a secured pathway to college and limited workforce outcomes.

It is time to stop sanctioning inequity and start serving equity in special education, for Black students with special needs in particular. We can remove *Racialized Educational Disability Injustices (REDI)* (because of poverty, hate, and ignorance), with anti-racist practices and policies that are research-based and cost-effective. *Pour the Water: Transformative Solutions for Equity and Justice in Special Education* demands that Goal 4 be realized as, *a specific prioritization in removing the barriers caused by racialized educational disability injustices in early childhood through secondary education for Black students with special education needs because of giftedness, disabilities, and medical conditions.*

Introduction

Are you Ready?

Are you ready to remove Racialized Educational Disability Injustices (REDI)? To start, we must be *REAL*:

- (R) Reveal: We must reveal our reality and wrestle with some uncomfortable topics and reasoning.
- (E) Equity-minded: We must be equity-minded to go beyond equalized education.
- (A) Align: We must align student needs with appropriate and accessible learning.
- (L) Leverage: We must leverage clear and legal language to level the education field for greater access and engagement.

If you are ready to be REAL, declare your mission readiness: *"I am ready to remove Racialized Educational Disability Injustices (REDI)."*

The frameworks presented in this text are designed to level the playing field and place educational leadership equity into the hands of parents and practitioners who seek success for Black children with special needs and/or disabilities. This text is written for parents, professionals, and policymakers with the hope that they will embrace data, experiences, and strategies for improving the educational experience of every Black student with special needs, further known as BSSN. Like Marian Wright-Edelman, I oppose grammar rules to lower the case for "Black" and "White."

One goal is to develop a common language so parents, professionals, and policymakers can share the accountability for understanding and implementing change. It is my hope that policymakers will recognize the roles of professionals, parents will understand the perspectives of professionals, and professionals will respect the parents' positions. About disproportionality and its causes and solutions, with *Pour the Water: Transformative Solutions for Equity & Justice in Special Education*, these stakeholders can, in the words of bell hooks, "....take that abstraction and articulate (it) in a language that renders it accessible—not less complex or rigorous—but simply more accessible" (bell hooks, 1989, p. 30).

Get Set...

While students receive free public education in the U.S., PreK is not universally free, and quality of services from general education to its partners, special education and gifted education, is not equitable for all students. The percentage of the U.S.'s seven million students in public special education varies across states, averaging around 15%. Black, Indigenous, and Latinx students with Special Needs (BILSSN), are 17%, 19%, and 14% respectively, of the total students serviced under the IDEA (Individuals with Disabilities Education Act). Special education is highly valuable. For Black student however, it is laden with identification errors, inappropriate services, lack of meaningful progress, and infidelity of interventions.

Students are identified and receive services under IDEA for a range of disabilities: Specific Learning Disability (SLD) being the highest at 26% and Hearing Impairment (HI) at 1%, the lowest. Accurate identification leads to appropriate services under IDEA, and there is a significant under-identification of Black students. According to the American Academy of Pediatrics, from kindergarten to eighth grade, children of the Black race are five times less likely than children of the White race to be diagnosed and serviced by IDEA (Morgan et al., 2013). This under-identification (and misidentification) continues through secondary education and is also related to service inequities. As does global illiteracy, special education service inequity contributes to an inevitable course of lifelong limitations for those students and their families who are already plagued by persistent barriers.

Systemic racism has made disparity in special education commonplace. Policies, practices, and research to support special education equity do exist. In this text, research and insights from a variety of sources are referenced, with clarity and context. Included is data from United States

Introduction

Commission on Civil Rights GAO (Government Accountability Office) reports, research from universities such as Pennsylvania State University, guidance from COPAA (Council of Parents, Advocates and Attorneys), examples from states such as Maryland State Department of Education, and many other agencies, institutes, and programs. Perspectives through interviews and direct statements from politicians, practitioners, and experts are also included to provide the appropriate contexts and effective solutions for disparity and disproportionality.

Representative Bobby Scott, Chairman of the Committee on Education and Labor, released a statement on the 2019 Government Accountability Office (GAO) report on Special Education IDEA. He stated: "The data clearly show that the civil rights protections provided under the Individuals with Disabilities Education Act are not equally accessible to all students." (Scott, 2019) Beyond supporting this position, the text also highlights the under-identification of Black students with special needs and how to equitably implement solutions.

Pour the Water: Transformative Solutions for Equity &Justice in Special Education is a resource to inform stakeholders, consultants, and leadership on special education equity for Black students with special needs. The text presents testimonies, identifies policies and available resources, recalls key factors of disproportionality, and shows parents, teachers, service providers, administrators, and community leaders how they too can make a difference for gifted or disabled Black children labeled.

Pour the Water: Transformative Solutions for Equity and Justice in Special Education:

- will not conclude that special education is detrimental,
- will hold general education accountable for inclusion,
- will show proper identification is necessary to address disproportionality and the school-to-prison pipeline, and

- will help parents and professionals apply benefits from IDEA and Free and Appropriate Public Education (FAPE).

Pour the Water: Transformative Solutions for Equity & Justice in Special Education was written for several stakeholders. For example, Black mothers particularly have a longstanding history of heartache experiencing the denial of their child's potential. Hebraist and Torah Teacher, Moreh Mayim, says that the word for mother in ancient Hebrew, is *Amma*, and shows that she is the "glue" of the household. In other words, she holds it all together: Preparing for IEP meetings, speaking up and asking questions, helping with homework, talking with teachers and staff, and preparing a home environment conducive to learning success. Thus, she feels deep personal disappointment when she is unable to hold her house together. This disappointment is the pain you see in her face during IEP meetings and the sorrow in her eyes when prison becomes her child's new home.

By embracing the practices outlined, stakeholders will lessen Black mothers' pain and cries…

- at the doctor's office, when they hear the diagnosis.
- at home, because their child is failing academically.
- at school, during the IEP meetings when denied services.
- at work, wondering if their child is okay at school.
- at night, because their child is involved in unlawful acts.
- at prison, seeing their child inside the visitation site room.

We need to begin with compassion for these mothers and have passion for equity and justice, ready to remove Racialized Educational Disability Injustice (REDI).

Introduction

Go!

The double inequity of racialized bias and special needs oversight has lit a fire under a growing number of parents, educators, and professionals to learn how to bring accountability for millions of children with disabilities who are denied access to equitable education and opportunities to discover and meet their potential. *Pour the Water Transformative Solutions for Equity & Justice in Special Education* gives you the practical changes you can make today to reach our preschoolers, redirect our middle schoolers, and refer our high schoolers to productive postsecondary resources, before they enter the prison or cycle of poverty.

Chapter 1 summarizes the development of the U.S. public school system and the emergence of qualifications for and regulations about special education services for students with disabilities. *Chapter 2* gives context to the students we seek to serve, illuminating the characteristics, challenges, and crises of our peculiar treasures: Black, Indigenous, and Latinx child learners. *Chapter 3* introduces us to a character named James and explores the data showing disproportionality and the school-to-prison pipeline. *Chapter 4* introduces us to a BSSN and explores disparities in outcomes. *Chapters 5 through 9* describe essential strategies that form the acronym *SEE US*.

- *S*ynchronize Health & Education: Helping physicians and parents reckon with identification, stigma, and treatment.

- *E*ducational Leadership for Parents© & Professionals: Encouraging and equipping parents to navigate their child's education.

- *E*quity through Prioritization: Uncomfortable and necessary strategies to level the learning field.

- *U*niversal Design for Learning & Accessibility: Research-based practices that are beneficial to all students.

- *S*pecial Education Advocacy: Guidance on forming an expert, unbiased opinion on the needs of the child.

Chapter 10 provides added reflection and a way forward with new stakeholder recommendations. The appendices include a glossary of terms, interviews with key pioneers in special education equity, and other resources of interest to the reader. Stakeholders who commit to antiracist policies, effective practices, and proper pedagogy will enhance services, instruction, and advocacy for Black students with special needs.

The title, *Pour the Water,* equates water with education. As essential as water is to the body, education is to the mind. *Pour the Water* is a demand that critical resources be streamed to benefit Black students with special needs. The cover graphic illustrates water as if educational resources were poured out directly onto the mind of the Black student with special needs. The value of the text and its applications is to see the alignment of resources by way of a plumbline to benefit Black students with special needs for postsecondary opportunities, rather than the pipeline that transports unlearned Black students to prison.

WRITTEN TESTIMONIAL

This book offers an abundance of data about how educational systems fail to prepare Black students with the skills to succeed in life. The disparities you point out are glaring. Even more important, the book offers solutions to overcoming what continues to be a lack of equity and justice that leads to over-identification or failing to educate Black students with special needs. I think the theme that prevails throughout this book is how an educational system works to benefit Whites to the disadvantage of the BSSN and constantly reminds the reader of how vitally important it is to support parents of Black students with special needs. The research data you share throughout the book demonstrates that a child's race and ethnicity is related to the high probability of being inappropriately identified as a student being intellectually disabled or emotionally disturbed.

Introduction

The heart of the book is chapters 5-9. Each of the introductory goals is written like an IEP goal for the student; however the goal is written for the system. By starting each chapter with a goal for the system, the focus is on what the overall educational system and other organizations need to do to address the issues of inequity and injustice for BSSNs. Having this type of goal at the beginning of the chapter serves as a map to help focus and implement the recommendations and measure the success or failure of the goal(s).

The model of working on each individual chapter for a month is really the essential guide for how this book can be used within school systems, university training programs, and other organizations whose purpose is to improve a continuum of services for BSSNs that are not being appropriately identified or receiving the services they need for life. This plan also demonstrates that BSSNs have continued to experience persistent systematic oppression experienced over hundreds of years in America, which one is clearly reminded of through every chapter in the book.

The concluding chapter offers suggestions for planning and implementing these goals.

—Robert J. Felton
Education Consultant, Weinfeld Education Group

Chapter 1

Perspectives on Education History

Funding and facilitation for educational accessibility and appropriateness for Black and all public school students with disabilities and medical conditions is the responsibility of the Office of Special Education Programs (OSEP) within the United States Department of Education. The U.S. Department of Education was formalized as a cabinet agency in 1867 to administer Pre-K-12 education. However, in 1868 it was demoted to an Office of Education due to concern that the Department would exercise too much control over local schools. During the 1960s, Johnson's War on Poverty sought an expansion of federal funding for education, and in 1979 the current Department of Education came into being (U.S. Department of Education, 2018).

The school system as we know it today was influenced by the vision of Horace Mann. In the nineteenth and twentieth centuries, immigrant populations grew exponentially, and Americans feared that immigrants would bring unknown languages, hatred, crime, and intolerance into the country. Mann, an educational reformer, believed that educating children from different backgrounds in the same schools would fuel acceptance among the children and spur productive socialization to benefit the economy and condition of America. The education system has since assumed the responsibility to promote citizenry through character maturation and skills cultivation for self-sufficiency, family sustenance, and community interdependence. Schools model the greater society by fostering tolerance for differences (e.g., race, religion), and classrooms facilitate teacher-imposed expectations and student self-discipline.

Mann was an abolitionist who believed in the powers of faith in God and in the capacity of oppressed young men to achieve human freedom over human slavery. Mann borrowed his education vision from the Prussian model of free education, where the independent thinking of soldiers bore the blame for Prussia's loss to France in 1806 as the leader of the *War of the Fourth Coalition*. Education reform was Prussia's solution for a more efficient military; it emphasized academic rigor, centralization, and standardization. In addition, Prussia sought to educate children on four core principles of civic duty: discipline, respect for authority, and, most notably, the ability to follow orders. Even the Prussian (and subsequent American education model) was not a novel concept. Loyalist teaching was the premise of education in ancient Egypt for the Pharaoh.

Impact of Oppression

By 1890, thousands of children were learning manual trades, and the early special education programs focused on the "moral training" of Black students. Part of the socialization mechanism by the early Europeans was to train Blacks to be as productive as possible for service (Wrightslaw.com, 2021). In 1895, the South Carolina constitution added literacy tests as qualifications for enfranchisement. Author Ta-Nehisi Coates describes in his book, *We Were Eight Years in Power*, ". . .when those measures proved insufficient to enforcing white supremacy, Black citizens were shot, tortured, beaten and maimed" (Coates, 2017).

The brutal and cruel practice of chattel slavery of Blacks in America beginning in 1619 left descendants educationally, emotionally, and culturally devastated, yet surprisingly spiritually resilient for dozens of generations afterwards. In the eighteenth and nineteenth centuries, enslaved Blacks developed secret schools amidst literacy bans. Many Blacks were beaten or killed if they were found able to read. Around 1865 enslaved Blacks emerged out of slavery, and the Freedmen's Bureau Act of 1865 provisioned freed Blacks (and White refugees) who were destitute of critical resources such as food, clothing, and schools to pursue life, liberty, and happiness. Both formerly enslaved Blacks and freed Blacks (Freedmen) quested for a free mindset and an education of self-sufficiency, work skills, artisanry, and design. Blacks developed labor schools during the early twentieth century, and citizenship schools were formed in the 1950s. Before then, Black schoolhouses were commonplace in communities across southern states as free, "safe spaces" for Blacks to gain their own academic footing, develop resilient character, and learn trade skills.

The early Europeans, under the authority of the United States, slaughtered and subjugated Indigenous Americans. The depletion of indigenous-stewarded natural resources, culture, and community poisoned their prosperity and potential. Native Americans valued education through community storytelling, culture, spiritual appreciation, and apprenticeship. Unfortunately, according to the White House,

> *Beginning with the Indian Civilization Act of 1819, federally run Indian boarding schools were used to culturally assimilate Native American children who were forcibly removed from their families and communities and relocated to distant residential facilities where their Native identities, languages, traditions, and beliefs were forcibly suppressed. The conditions in these schools were usually harsh, and sometimes abusive and deadly.*

Due to the influence of Spanish culture in Mexico, Native Mexicans have a long history of Catholic education. However, coupled with widespread poverty and poor public school facilities, new laws restricting Spanish made schooling unavailable for most Mexican children in the state (Velez, 1994), and the majority of Mexican migrant children never went beyond the primary grades in Texas (Warburton, Wood, & Crane, 1943). Students were placed in "Mexican-only classes," and schools were used to train Mexican Americans to be domestics and farmhands and occupy the manufacturing sector's lower rungs.

The OC: The Original Curriculum

Educator and author Harold Garnet Black stated that reading classics by authors such as Chaucer, Dickens, Emerson, and Poe, "widens one's horizon in a field of knowledge that invites still further exploration" (Black, 1947). Literature helps students experience character depth, change, and motivation. Character development has largely been exercised using literature in the mainstream school setting. Common reads include:

- *Of Mice and Men* (John Steinbeck)
- *The Grapes of Wrath* (John Steinbeck)
- *To Kill a Mockingbird* (Harper Lee)
- *The Bluest Eye* (Toni Morrison)
- *Their Eyes Were Watching God* (Zora Neale Hurston)
- *Night* (Ellie Wiesel)

I also remember reading character-shaping books like:

- *Black Boy* (Richard Wright)
- *Charlotte's Web* (E.B. White)
- *Uncle Tom's Cabin* (Harriet Beecher Stowe)
- *Nigger: An Autobiography* (Dick Gregory)

All these books offered new perspectives and gave shape to personal choice-making. William Shakespeare's writings have long been revered both for their depth of character development and human exploration.

Black also advocated for the English Bible to be included in American schools' literary source lists. Black describes the Bible's value as a "spiritual guide, (for) the profound knowledge of human nature it displays, (and) its sheer literary merit," which has been, "proclaimed by thousands of writers, statesmen, and educational leaders." (Black, 1947). Throughout history, the Bible (e.g. Torah, Septuagint), has been widely cited for its laws and moral code on how people should treat each other. According to Black, the earliest school training in Puritan New England "had a distinctly religious basis." For example, children were taught to "associate each letter with some biblical story, name or event" through the New England Primer (first published in 1688 by Benjamin Harris), also known as "The Little Bible" (Black, 1947).

During the early colonial period of the seventeenth century (influenced largely by religious beliefs and legal conflicts), Black says that it was the "aim of the schools to teach children to read the Bible" and colleges to train men for ministry. The founding fathers often used "virtue," a high-frequency biblical word defined as the conformity to a standard of right (Webster's Dictionary), describing its moral standard as the "necessary fountainhead of a free society" as cited by the National Center for Constitutional Studies (Stedman & Lewis, 1987). Benjamin Franklin, who is arguably America's key Founding Father wrote, "I think with you, that nothing is of more importance for the public weal, than to form and train up youth in wisdom and virtue" (Letter to Samuel Johnson, August 23, 1750). Undoubtedly, his appeal for society's morality had its origin in the verse from Proverbs, the Bible's book of wisdom and virtue: "Train up a child in the way he should go, and when he is old he will not depart from it" (Proverbs 22:6 KJV).

Franklin continued in his letter to Samuel Johnson:

I think also, that general virtue is more probably to be expected and obtained from the education of youth, than from the exhortation of adult persons; bad habits and vices of the mind, being, like diseases of the body, more easily prevented than cured. I think moreover that talents for the education of youth are the gift of God; and that he on whom they are bestowed, whenever a way is opened for the use of them, is as strongly called as if he heard a voice from heaven: Nothing more surely pointing out duty in a public service, than ability and opportunity of performing it. (National Archives, 1961)

After the Revolutionary War, religious education waned. According to the Christian Science Monitor, "both black and white schools continued a conservative Evangelical Protestant teaching of the Bible through the end of World War II" (Marquand, 1985). While the schoolhouses for Blacks and Whites were separate in the South, their curricula used the same book: the Bible. In Virginia, it is believed that "as many as five percent of enslaved people may have been literate by the start of the American Revolution (1775–1783)" with their education tied to religious conversion and instruction (Encyclopedia Virginia, 2023). "Literate enough to read a catechism", was the goal and "many enslavers viewed Christian teaching as their duty…" (Encyclopedia Virginia, 2023). "Nor is the slave by such prohibition cut off from learning the doctrines of Christianity…for negroes to attend Divine worship, and be instructed" (O'Neall, 1848).

Slave owners used the Bible as a double-edged sword, a razor-sharp instrument carefully crafted to control their chattel slaves. According to the Museum of the Bible, in the U.S., *The Slave Bible* had only 232 of the 1189 chapters available to forbidden readers. Specifically, 90% of the Old Testament was redacted, including the entire book of Exodus, which is the blueprint for freedom, and Jeremiah, which would have condemned work without pay. Also missing was 50% of the New Testament, including the entire book of Galatians, which provided forbidden commentary on slavery.

Reading and writing and its subsequent literacies were banned for the enslaved to prevent ideas of freedom and concepts of hope. Any enslaved caught reading or writing resulted in whipping and the dismembering of hands and other body parts (Span, 2005). South Carolina was the first colony to enact Anti-literacy laws in 1740 after the Stono Rebellion of 1739 (the largest uprising of the enslaved), making teaching literacy punishable by 100 British pounds and six months in prison (Span, 2005).

Excerpt from South Carolina Act of 1740:

> CHATTELS *are not educated! And if human beings are to be held in chattel hood, education must be withheld from them.*
>
> *Whereas, the having slaves taught to write, or suffering them to be employed in writing, may be attended with great inconveniences; Be it enacted, that all and every person and persons whatsoever, who shall hereafter teach or cause any slave or slaves to be taught to write, or shall use or employ any slave as a scribe, in any manner of writing whatsoever, hereafter taught to write, every such person or persons shall, for every such offense, forfeit the sum of one hundred pounds, current money. (The American Slave Code, Chapter VI)*

It was also an "unlawful assembly" to gather at schools or other place to read or write (Virginia Revised Code of 1819). Insurrectionist, Nat Turner defied the anti-literacy laws and was learned in the Bible among other skills. According to the *Confessions of Nat Turner to Thomas Gray*, he was gifted and could read at a young age without being trained in the alphabet. Gray said of his confession, "As to his ignorance, he certainly never had the advantages of education, but he can read and write, (it was taught him by his parents), and for natural intelligence and quickness of apprehension, is surpassed by few men I have ever seen." According to Turner, "the Spirit appeared..." and inspired him in 1831 to lead a revolt against slavery in a Virginia town then called Jerusalem, Southampton, where 51 White men, women, and children were slaughtered. (Breen, 2020). Remarkable that a child with such gifts would be bound by shackles, only to be loosed to violence.

As Union armies arrived in Virginia in 1861, African Americans immediately began opening schools. They utilized Black teachers and, over the years, an increasing number of White Northerners. Around the time of the Civil War, literacy rose from about 10% to 30% for Blacks, and by 1910, it was at 70%. The enslaved had a burning desire to read, write, and become learned that can only be compared to that burning bush on Mount Sinai. The bush burned with fire and could not be consumed or extinguished.

And there was always an insatiable desire to learn. Booker T. Washington in his book, *Up From Slavery*, recalled an elderly woman who, "hobbled into the room where I was, leaning on a cane. She was clad in rags; but they were clean. She said:

> *'Mr. Washin'ton, God knows I spent de bes' days of my life in slavery. God knows I's ignorant an' poor… I knows you is tryin' to make better men an' better women for de coloured race. I ain't got no money, but I wants you to take dese six eggs, what I's been savin' up, an' I wants you to put dese six eggs into the eddication of dese boys an' gals." (Washington, 1901)*

The System Design Thinking

The first Department of Education in 1867 was created to collect data, promote education, and appropriate land for reservation schools. It was not to decide on matters such as teacher qualifications, curriculum, or even accommodations for students with disabilities as it does today. However, the questions of community school education quality, the race for global competition, the demands for science and workforce readiness, and war implications such as mothers entering into the workforce spurred the common school or public school movement, and the Department of Education we have today formed in 1979.

The special education system is under the umbrella of the greater education system and must be recognized, legitimized and adequately subsidized. Students must qualify for special education services to warrant services allocated by the school district, which also funds general education. As well, students must maximize their response to interventions and establish behavior patterns over time, essential enough for the system to regard them as eligible for its resources. These are some examples of the factors within the current special education system. In a 2018 report and 2023 review of the State Systemic Improvement Plans by the National Center for Learning Disabilities, states reveal capacity challenges for such practices as, Universal Design for Learning, the inclusion of parent and student voice, integration of effective collaboration, strategic allocation of resources, alignment with state priorities, implementation and measurement of results, cooperation between special education and general education, and "conditions for continuous improvement to advance educational equity" (OSEP, 2024).

For BSSNs, the process to qualify for services is a fundamental flaw in a system where there are already related hurdles. While the Child Find identification process is supposed to find them, BSSN parents spend an enormous amount of energy trying to find education services for their child with a gift, delay, disability or difference. Being disenfranchised from societal resources at large, and then having to navigate a legal process within a common education system is counterintuitive.

Another flaw in the special education system for BSSNs is that the system operates with its own inputs. The same system which defines deviance, also defines personality, defines intelligence, and determines norms or what is normal. Departed educational psychologist, Amos Wilson, describes this system as "maintaining the constant" of the political and economic production agenda. Progress is unattained and qualifications remain systemically unmatched which is pertinent to what he says is the "slavery economy", with the intention on retaining slave-like labor. Before the 1950s, the dominant view toward this group (Blacks) involved educating them not for equal citizenship but for lower-ranked positions they would hold (Skiba et al., 2008).

I interviewed Dr. Walter Dunson, author and reading expert for over 30 years, on his observations and reflections; his master's thesis was on the public education school model. Here is one of the many significant points he made:

> *The entire educational system here in the United States is designed to replicate the social divisions of labor where you have two different tracks, just like you have two different tracks of labor where you have the management track, and you have the working class. So you have that type of school structure designed to keep people or to place people on the management track and those designed to place people working in the working man line. For example, I have taught in a lot of private schools and I have taught in public schools. The immediate difference is sound. In private schools, there are no bells, no alarms—when classes are over, it's see you tomorrow, kids get up, and they head out. In the public schools, everything is regimented. Bells alarms dang ding dang, and it replicates working in a factory; I mean, it literally does.*

In *Pedagogy of the Oppressed,* Paolo Freire, a renowned Brazilian anti-oppressionist, makes it clear that the narrative character of education is an oppressive instrument designed and delivered to guide the thoughts, intentions, and actions of others (Jackson, 2018).

An Integrated Timeline of Disability and Race in Education

In the 1940s, programs for children with learning disabilities became common. Most special education took place within the home, or private residential programs. Yet for most with disabilities, special education programs were unavailable. Programs for learning disabilities (referred to as "brain injury" and "minimal brain dysfunction,") became more common in the 1940's (Wrightslaw.com, 2022).

1948 United Nations Universal Declaration on Human Rights

The U.N. Declaration on Human Rights provided an expectation for human freedom and opportunity in America and around the globe. "Everyone has the right to life, liberty, and security of person. No one shall be held in slavery or servitude; slavery and the slave trade shall be prohibited in all their forms." According to the U.N. Universal Declaration of Human Rights, "All human beings are born free and equal in dignity and rights. They are endowed with reason and conscience and should act toward one another in a spirit of brotherhood." Article 5 stated, "No one shall be subjected to torture or cruel, inhuman or degrading treatment or punishment." In 2008, then-U.N. Secretary-General Ban Ki-Moon, at the Commemoration of the International Day of Remembrance of the Victims of Slavery and the Transatlantic Slave Trade, proclaimed that "considering the enormous historic proportions and impact, it is a cruel irony that little is known about the slave trade." He said:

> *That is why today is so important. We must remember and honor those who spent their lives as slaves, who were defined under laws as nothing more than chattel, property, and real estate, who were essentially treated not as humans but as "things." (KI-Moon, 2008)*

Ban Ki-Moon essentially said how cruel it is not to remember slavery's cruelty. Cambridge defines cruelty as "unnecessary harm or punishment," and the Book of Proverbs says that "wrath is cruel" (27:4). It further illustrates that "a righteous (man) regardeth the life of his beast, but the compassion (tender mercies) of the wicked are cruel" (12:10). Remembering the monstrous brutality and sacrifices of a tortured people is a modest act of compassion.

1954 Integration: Schools Become Integrated by Law

On May 17, 1954, the U.S. Supreme Court unanimously ruled that racial segregation in public schools violated the 14th Amendment to the Constitution, which says that no state may deny equal protection of the laws to anyone within its jurisdiction. The 1954 decision declared that separate educational facilities were inherently unequal. Following a series of Supreme Court cases argued between 1938 and 1950 that chipped away at legalized segregation, Brown v. Board of Education of Topeka reversed an earlier Supreme Court ruling (Plessy v. Fergus, 1896) that permitted "separate but equal" public facilities. The 1954 decision was limited to public schools, but it was believed to imply that segregation was not permissible in other public facilities. Chief Justice Warren delivered the following opinion (excerpt) of the Court:

> *It (education) is the very foundation of good citizenship. Today it is a principal instrument in awakening the child to cultural values, in preparing him for later professional training, and in helping him to adjust normally to his environment. In these days, it is doubtful that any child may reasonably be expected to succeed in life if he is denied the opportunity of an education. Such an opportunity, where the state has undertaken to provide it, is a right which must be made available to all on equal terms.* (National Archives)

The opinion supported that "To separate them from others of similar age and qualifications solely because of their race generates a feeling of inferiority as to their status in the community that may affect their hearts and minds in a way unlikely ever to be undone" It also cited that "Segregation of white and colored children in public schools has a detrimental effect upon the colored children", especially where segregation is sanctioned by the law. The ruling concluded that, "Segregation with the sanction of law, therefore, has a tendency to [retard] the educational and mental development of negro children and to deprive them of some of the benefits they would receive in a racial[ly] integrated school system" (Brown v. Board of Education, National Archives). See the end of the chapter for a related discussion question.

Support for school integration was not unanimous across the Black communities. A 1973 Gallup poll indicated that "18% of the nation opposed public school integration"; 19% were White and 9% Black (New York Times, 1973). Parents and policymakers had concerns over busing students outside of their communities into an unfamiliar Black or White community to attend integrated schools. Almost half of the respondents preferred changes in neighborhood boundaries or the development of affordable housing in middle-class neighborhoods, rather than busing to fulfill integration. In 1975, then-Senator Joe Biden opposed forced integration. He said, "I think the concept of busing ... that we are going to integrate people so that they all have the same access and they learn to grow up with one another and all the rest, is a rejection of the whole movement of black pride, is a rejection of the entire black awareness concept where black is beautiful, black culture should be studied, and the cultural awareness of the importance of their own identity, their own individuality" (NPR, 1975).

There was some reluctance to desegregation among Black communities. Justice Warren's ruling from the SCOTUS was premised that unequal access to White schools and facilities hindered the motivation and learning of Black children. They would feel inferior based upon the denial to collaborate with White children and access the buildings, curricula, qualifications, and teacher salaries which were unequal. While the facilities of Negro Schools could be classified as inferior, the sovereignty factor of those schools was valued and defended by a few. Some Black citizens recognized that integration would result in the loss of Negro schools. In *Along Freedom Road: Hyde County, North Carolina, and the Fate of Black Schools in the South:*

> *For an entire year, 1968 through 1969, in North Carolina's Hyde County, the county's Black citizens refused to send their children to school in protest of a desegregation plan that required closing two historically Black schools in their remote coastal community. Parents and students held nonviolent protests daily for five months, marched twice on the state capital in Raleigh, and drove the Ku Klux Klan out of the county in a massive gunfight. (Cecelski, 2016)*

Along with the increase in integrated academics, the establishment of Black schools, and the emergence of disproportionately followed desegregation. After the decision in *Brown vs. Board of Education*, parents began bringing lawsuits against schools for excluding children with disabilities. At the end of this chapter, see Pinellas County Schools District and Maryland State in the Spotlight as examples of post-integration outcomes.

1964

The Freedom Schools of the 1960s were part of a long line of efforts to liberate people from oppression by using the tool of popular education. Over the Freedom Summer of 1964, more than 40 Freedom Schools were set up in black communities throughout Mississippi. The purpose was to try to end the political displacement of African Americans by encouraging students to become active citizens and socially involved within the community. Over 3,000 African American students attended these schools in the summer of 1964 (Menkart et al., 2018).

The Black independent school movement came on the heels of a largely failed push for substantive integration. As it became clear that the federal and state implementation of post-Brown integration orders had little effect on the majority of Black students who were still trapped in highly segregated, under-resourced, and academically substandard schools, community members shifted their focus to gaining control over their local schools (New York Times, 1999). When this movement for community control met staunch resistance from teachers and administrators, the Black community, influenced by the era's burgeoning emphasis on Black pride and cultural consciousness, turned their attention toward developing autonomous institutions.

Independent Freedom schools embraced research-based practices such as high academic standards, cultural affirmation, and personalized attention. In his manuscript for independent education, Black power, and radical imagination, historian Russell Rickford describes the value of these independent schools. In his words,

> *Pan-African nationalist schools were far more than vessels of formal education. They were cooperatives, collectives, cultural centers, organs of community action, and laboratories for a spectrum of ideas—from*

anti-imperialism and Third Worldism on the left to patriarchy and racial fundamentalism on the right. (Rickford, 2016)

1965 Elementary and Secondary Education Act (ESSA)

Congress enacted the Elementary and Secondary Education Act (ESSA) in 1965. The ESSA supplies a means to help ensure that disadvantaged students can access quality education. Many children with disabilities were denied access to education and opportunities to learn. Under ESSA, states must administer an annual, summative assessment to capture student achievement in English/Language Arts, Mathematics, and Science for use in accountability plans and to meet transparency reporting requirements. Widespread cancellation of testing in Spring 2020 due to school impact from the COVID-19 pandemic was the first time a nationwide assessment waiver had been issued since the passage of the landmark education law. The ESSA was amended in 1966 to establish a program that would assist states in the "initiation, expansion, and improvement of programs and projects... for the education of handicapped children." According to WrightsLaw.com, "Neither program included any specific mandates on the use of the funds... nor could either program be shown to have significantly improved the education of children with disabilities" (WrightsLaw.com, 1999).

1970 Education of the Handicapped Act

In 1970, U.S. schools educated only one in five children with disabilities, and many states had laws excluding certain students, including children who were deaf, blind, emotionally disturbed, or had an intellectual disability. The Education of the Handicapped Act replaced ESSA in 1970, aiming to help states develop educational programs and resources for students with disabilities.

1973 Section 504 of the Rehabilitation Act

Section 504 provides that:

No otherwise qualified individual with a disability in the United States... shall, solely by reason of her or his disability, be excluded from the participation in, be denied the benefits of, or be subjected to discrimination under any program or activity receiving Federal financial assistance... (Duncan, 2010) (Free appropriate public education under section 504)

1975 Education for all Handicapped Children (EHA)

Congress enacted Public Law 94-142 in 1975. This act required all public schools accepting federal funds to provide equal access to education for children with physical and mental disabilities. Also known as the EHA, this law supports states and localities in protecting the rights of, meeting the individual needs of, and improving the results for infants, toddlers, children, and youth with disabilities and their families. Mainly, Congress found an overrepresentation of minority children noting that poor African American children were overrepresented in special education. Public Law 94-142 was a landmark law and was the original name of the Individuals with Disabilities Education Act, or IDEA, renamed in a 1990 reauthorization. The law was last reauthorized in 2004, and the Department has periodically issued new or revised regulations to address the implementation and interpretation of the IDEA.

Beginning as early as the mid-1970s, many independent Black schools faced many problems that made it difficult for many to survive. Independent institutions faced external threats from government-sponsored sabotage and internal threats posed by members of the Black community suffering from the effects of systemic racism and immorality, such as economic decline, unemployment, and drug abuse. Other sources of internal strife included ideological and political conflicts, physical burn-out, and financial collapse. According to the African American Intellectual History Society's (AAIHS) Charter Schools and the Black Independent School Movement, these issues were further compounded by parents who began to favor traditional education over cultural development, emphasizing social participation and economic competition (Rickford, 2017) Overall, the independent school movement reached an irresolvable impasse on where charter schools fit within the struggle for Black nationalist liberation. While the charter system has allowed some former independent Black institutions to remain open and continue to serve their communities, it remains to be seen if the sacrifices outweigh the benefits.

By 2002, the National Research Council had validated that a "... child's race and ethnicity are significantly related to the probability that he or she will be inappropriately identified as disabled." (National Academies, 2002).

2004 Individuals with Disabilities Education Act (IDEA)

Congress has amended and renamed the special education law several times since 1975. On December 3, 2004, the Individuals with Disabilities Education Act was amended again. The reauthorized statute is the Individuals with Disabilities Education Improvement Act of 2004, known as IDEA 2004. The statute is in Volume 20 of the United States Code (USC), beginning at Section 1400. The special education regulations are published in Volume 34 of the Code of Federal Regulations (CFR) beginning in Section 300. In reauthorizing IDEA, Congress increased the focus on accountability and improved outcomes by emphasizing reading, early intervention, and research-based instruction by requiring that special education teachers be highly qualified (Wrightslaw.com, 2023).

Purpose of Individuals with Disabilities Act (IDEA)

The Individuals with Disabilities Education Act of 2004 has two primary purposes according to Wrightslaw.com. First, is to provide an education that meets a child's unique needs and prepares the child for further education, employment, and independent living. Second, it is to protect the rights of children with disabilities and their parents (Wrightslaw.com). Congress increased focus on accountability and improved outcomes and instruction by requiring special education teachers to be highly qualified. Congress emphasized aligning IDEA 2004 with the No Child Left Behind. The Individualized Education Plan (IEP) is an essential instrument of IDEA.

Free and Appropriate Public Education (FAPE)

Free and Appropriate Public Education (FAPE) is the strong arm of IDEA, in providing for students with disabilities. According to the U.S. Department of Education, as cited on its website:

> *Section 504 and Title II require public schools to provide appropriate education and modifications, aids and related services free of charge to students with disabilities and their parents or guardians. The "appropriate" component means that this education must be designed to meet the individual educational needs of the student as determined through appropriate evaluation and placement procedures. However, students with disabilities must be educated with students without disabilities to the maximum extent appropriate. (Office of Civil Rights, 2013)*

Disproportionality

In the findings of IDEA 2004, Congress described ongoing problems with over-identifying minority children, including mislabeling and high dropout rates. Findings included the following: (1) more significant efforts are needed to prevent the intensification of problems connected with mislabeling and high dropout rates among minority children with disabilities; (2) more minority children continue to be served in special education than would be expected from the percentage of minority students in the general school population; (3) African American children are identified as having mental retardation and emotional disturbance at rates greater than their White counterparts. In the 1998–1999 school year, African American children represented just 14.8% of the population aged at six through 21 but comprised 20.2% of all children with disabilities; and (4) studies have found that schools with predominantly White students and teachers have placed disproportionately high numbers of their minority students into special education (Public Law 108-446 Section 601(c), Findings).

Disproportionality in identification among Black and White students was and is a disheartening condition of systemic racism. The National Research Council had already validated high probability that race and ethnicity were linked to overidentification of disability (2002). In 2015, Every Student Succeeds Act (ESSA), was reauthorized by President Obama in December, though without some parts pertaining to accountability-including the requirement for highly qualified teachers. In 2016, then U.S. Secretary of Education John King proclaimed, "Children with disabilities are often disproportionately and unfairly suspended and expelled from school and educated in classrooms separate from their peers." He said, "Children of color with disabilities are overrepresented within the special education population, and the contrast in how frequently they are disciplined is even starker." This chapter concludes with two school district spotlights on dis-proportionality.

2019

By the 2018-2019 school year, The U.S. had progressed from excluding nearly 1.8 million children with disabilities from public schools before EHA implementation to providing more than 7.5 million children with disabilities with special education and related services. In 2018-19, more than 64% of children with disabilities were in general education classrooms for 80% or more of their school day (IDEA Part B Child Count and Educational Environments Collection), and early intervention services were provided to more than 400,000 infants and toddlers with disabilities and their families (IDEA Part C Child Count and Settings). Despite this progress, the Government Accountability Office, November 2019, found that Black students are 40% more likely to be identified as having educational disabilities than their peers... and Black students are twice as likely to be identified as having emotional disturbance and intellectual disability as their peers. In addition, among families of students with disabilities, those with lower incomes and who have children of color are less likely than their affluent and White counterparts to access their legal rights under IDEA. In 2019, the U.S. Commission on

Civil Rights found that Black children with disabilities face an especially acute problem with being served appropriately, often subjected to disparate discipline punishment compared to their White, non-Hispanic peers.

Regrettably, even after the Brown vs. Board of Education (1954) decision, some educational practices, such as placing students in special education and sorting them by ability, separated minority students from others. In the 1960s and 1970s, court challenges occurred, contesting that discriminatory educational practices which led to the racial isolation of minority students were a violation of the Equal Protection Clause of the Constitution and Title VI of the Civil Rights Act of 1964. Although concerns about discriminatory practices led to research in the 1970s and 1980s, these early studies did not reveal insights into the mechanisms that promote racial differences in identifying students in special education. In later years, research focused more on the factors leading to this problem (Skiba et al., 2008).

2020

In June 2020, the U.S. Department of Education reported that most states failed education obligations to students with special needs. In addition, the global COVID-19 pandemic sent special needs students to home-based computers and services. As a result, several educators, professionals, and policymakers began sounding alarms (again) and exploring ways to make a difference.

One example of an effort is when Special Education Excellence for Underserved Students (SEE US) responded to the Maryland region's disproportionality using a strategy of equitable advocacy to collaborate with parents and school teams on behalf of Black students with special needs and to provide training and resources for professionals and stakeholders. I am the champion and coordinator of this initiative, and this book includes our story.

Spotlights

District Spotlight: Pinellas County Schools, Florida Disparity

After School Integration, statistical tracking for many districts and communities disclosed academic achievement gaps and discipline disparities between Black, Latinx, and White students. In 2010, Concerned Organization for Quality Education of Black Students, Inc. (COQEBS) became the court-approved entity to monitor and enforce the Pinellas County School Board's (PBS) commitment to providing quality education for Black students and holds accountable the District's Bridging the Gap (BTG) 10-year Plan (COQEBS Community Open Letter). In 2015 before the BTG, the PBS Graduation rate was 65% Black and 83% non-Black, and the discipline risk ratio was 2.3 for referrals and 4.3 for out-of-school suspensions for Black students; This meant that in 2021-2022, Black students were still two times and four times more likely than White students to be referred for discipline and receive out-of-school suspensions, respectively (PCSB, 2023).

Civil Rights attorneys familiar with the Pinellas County, Florida schools' disparities pointed out that desegregation is not just about Black students attending school with White students. They said, "It's about those Black students being treated fairly in those schools" (Weathers, 2020). According to Ricardo Davis, President of COQEBS, PBS has never had a Black or Hispanic Superintendent since its inception in 1912. (Powerbroker Magazine, 2022)

State Spotlight: Maryland State Department of Education Disproportionality

In 2023, Maryland submitted the results of a continuation study of a deep dive into data related to Maryland's children with disabilities (birth through 21 years) and the strategic response and programming of the Division of Early Intervention and Special Education Services. The study revealed significant disproportionality. Black/African American students disproportionately compose the students with disabilities at 39%, more than any other groups. Specific Learning Disability (26%) and Other Health Impairments (17%) were reported as the largest categories. Three local education agencies will be awarded grants to analyze the data and implement solutions, such as professional development.

Reflection Questions: Choose One or Both

Schools from four states (Kansas, South Carolina, Virginia, and Delaware), had argued that segregated public schools were unequal and did not provide equal protection of the laws. The Supreme Court decided that Black children had the right to equal education and that segregated schools had no place in the education system. Separating children from their peers due to race promotes a feeling of inferiority that may never be undone.

1. Do you agree with the Supreme Court's decision that segregated schools have no place in the education system?
Why?

2. Does school segregation promote a feeling of inferiority?
How?

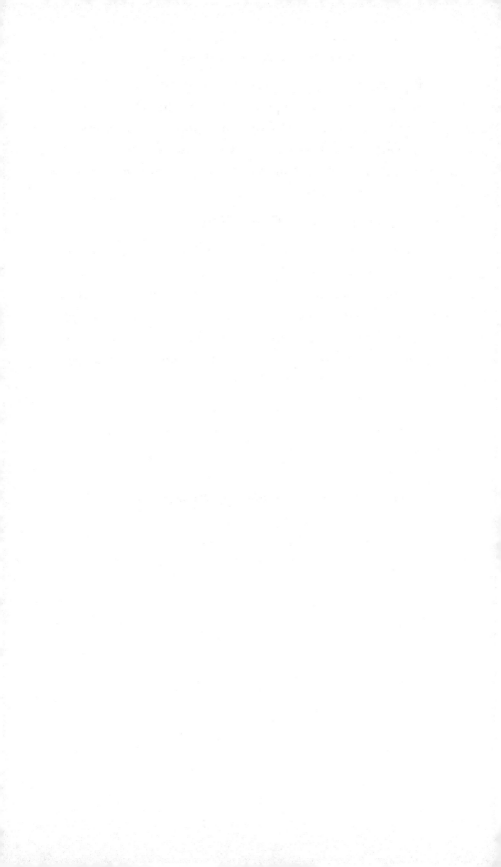

Chapter 2

Perspectives on Change in Systems, Practices, and People

The system in which we live, work, play, and love our families is creating economic and political productivity as intended; however, not to the benefit of everyone, but rather to the detriment of Black Students with Special Needs. This detriment is evidenced by their low academic achievement, the prevalence of poverty, and the highest incarceration rates.

Black children are rated to have the lowest opportunity to develop healthily. The Child Opportunity Index (COI) measures and maps 72,000 neighborhoods across the country on the quality of resources and conditions that matter for children (like early childhood education and schools) to develop healthily in the neighborhoods where they live. Nationally in 2021, the Child Opportunity Score (COS) for Black children is 24, Hispanic children 33, and White children 73. For example, in Maryland's Baltimore-Columbia-Towson metropolitan region where I was raised, the COS for Black children is cited as 53 points lower than White children. In Milwaukee, Wisconsin, the gap is 79 points: A typical Black child in Milwaukee is growing up in a neighborhood with a Child Opportunity Score of 6, whereas a White child's COS is 85. (Diversedatakids.org, 2022)

How we access resources makes a difference in the quality of life and, in our case, the quality of the educational experience. Multiple research studies demonstrate that a child's race and ethnicity are significantly related to the probability of being inappropriately identified as disabled.

We continue to see that disproportionality is due to "institutional racism, stereotypes, cultural incompetence, racial bias, and inequitable discipline policies" (Lehr & McComas, 2010). According to the Learning Disability Association, "Black students have been overrepresented in special education since the US Office of Civil Rights first started to sample school districts in 1968." Disparities in identification are most significant for specific learning disabilities (SLD), intellectual disabilities (ID), and emotional disturbances (ED). For example, black students are twice as likely to be labeled as emotionally disturbed and three times as likely to be identified with an ID compared to their White peers.

Disproportionality has several factors that should be considered with the contextual variables of the school. For example, you might find that the more students of color in a school, the greater the percentage of them who may be identified for special education services. Researchers have also suggested that teacher or assessment biases could have greater impact on the more subjective disabilities, leading to observed disparities. BSSNs are also disproportionately identified as having SLD. For example, during the 2013–14 school year BSSNs represented only 16% of the student population but 20% of students diagnosed with a specific learning disability.

Another factor is disparity in inclusion. Research has clearly shown the benefits of inclusion—the practice of educating special education students in general education classrooms alongside their peers who are not receiving special education services. When inclusion begins early, and embeds support into the curriculum, students have better outcomes, including higher test scores and graduation rates. However, once placed in special education, Black students are more likely to be taught in separate classrooms. While 55% of White students with disabilities spend more than 80% of their school day in a general education classroom, only a third of Black students spend that much time in a general education classroom.(MSDE, 2023)

It has been said that an ounce of prevention beats a pound of intervention. Since students of color already experience inequalities in schools at a high rate, the adverse outcomes associated with their misplacement in special education are serious. These outcomes include racial segregation, stigmatization, and group misrepresentation (Skiba et al., 2016). Given these conditions for BSSNs, we must encourage a focus on designing micro-systems of prevention and interventions that promote perspective change (Chapter 3), the RRIIPP (Chapter 4), and the SEEUS solutions (Chapters 5–9).

Seeing Transformation in Special Education

Special education, too, will see changes in referrals to disciplinary action and special education services. As you look for and participate in the system changes, be mindful of the basic principles of change. Change can happen instantly. The degrees and results of the change, however, take time. I have read many recommendations and white papers calling for changes in special education and discipline policies, warning that "changes do not occur overnight." While change results do not show overnight, in principle, change can occur as soon as you start to make a difference. When people resist change (or are in partnership with those who do), try to change too much or for too many at once, or are given permission to percolate passively, tolerance for deference can persist.

I do not anticipate an overhaul of the education system in the manner of a revolution where harmful practices change and are completely dismantled and rebuilt. However, efforts across policy, improvements in professional development, and greater engagement by parents and others will influence how BSSNs are served. We will want to see key signs of system success that will benefit the BSSN and their children across generations rather than changes that benefit societal systems and repeat cycles of oppression. If the shifts in special education are happening, there should be evidence of this direct, whole-child benefit.

Champions for BSSNs should look for signs in the classrooms and places where significant time is spent. While we wait for a seismic change or new system to change the outcomes, there are some interventions and strategies to employ specifically for BSSNs being taught in the home, learning pods, and public, private, and community schools. First, let us identify what we need to see, describe the premise of race and bias for why we need change, and summarize the systemic experience.

See Color

We tend to be acutely aware of our perceptions of others. We can sense confidence through the style of dress. We can hear ethnicity through language accents. We can see racial constructs through skin tone. Is it valuable to deny our eyesight and not see color? Perhaps we can reframe our thinking a bit. Let's recall two basic well-known principles: One, not all Black (nor are all Brown, nor are all White) people are of the same ethnicity; and two, all people look different because they are different. We are all unique beings with unique DNA, varying personalities, and even different tendencies toward disease, athleticism, and innovation, as just a few examples. Our outward visuals are mere abstracts of the diversity that lies beneath. But our country's history of racism based on color makes it necessary to see the color of our students and understand the legacy they have inherited.

The psychological legacy for BSSNs is one of resilience over generations, often fortified through a history of inhumane transatlantic travel, brutal enslavement and servitude, misappropriation of gifts and talents, and consistent subjection to substandard quality of services in America, like education. Our black students and their families have endured much, but that is not to say, however, that since they can endure, they should. See color for what it represents and go beyond to find what lies in each individual BSSN to develop their potential to transcend color connotations.

See Work

Raj Aggarwal, a former colleague and president of the social impact and racial equity marketing company, Provoc, once said, "Integrity is knowing the right thing to do and then doing it." What a powerful, yet practical principle; one that commands courage no matter how familiar it may be. Transforming how we support BSSNs to achieve the desired results outlined in this book is no light task, but the choice to see and do the work will define one's integrity. It is a heavy lift to accept the challenge and to work diligently and collectively toward those goals. You may have heard the saying, "The more you know, the more you ought to do," or to pull from one of Tionne Watkins (T-Boz of TLC) publicized quotes, "When you know better, you do better." Growing up in the 1970s and 80s we used to say, "Don't just talk about it; be about it." Whichever saying resonates with you best, the point is to focus on impact or outcomes, not intentions or plans.

See History

A marquee of oppression is diluted and misinformation, as Freire so illustratively articulates in *Pedagogy of the Oppressed*. Learn to see a 400-year timeline of development, culture, and relationships on the conflict between Black oppression and White supremacy in America from both points of view. Have empathy for the effects of slavery and systemic oppression on the relationships, development, and culture of your BSSNs. Additionally, exposure to the knowledge and relationship between racism and special education will awaken you to critically consider your role in the success of Black students with special needs. The application of identifying American history through the Black lens is empathetic.

The beginning of the experience of slavery for Blacks in America traded and sold from Africa was described during the first International Day of Remembrance for the Transatlantic Slave Trade.

> *Over more than four centuries, some 15 million Africans were taken from their homes across Africa and transported by force to the Americas. The number of people purchased by slave traders was even higher. Those enslaved people who survived were bought and sold, stripped of all dignity, and denied all human rights. Even their children could be taken from them and sold for the profit of their owners. The transatlantic slave trade remains a monstrous crime and a stain on human history. (UN Secretary-General, Ban Ki-Moon, 215)*

Literacy and freedom of thought were forbidden, leaving generations of Blacks without access to benefits that self-determination yielded for Whites and immigrants. After the abolition of slavery, amidst harsh racism and oppression, community-based education and home learning were administered before school integration. While the desegregation of schools was a landmark, its engagement dismantled the Black education community. Parents, teachers, and students were embedded right back under the thumb of an oppressive order, this time by choice.

See Through the "R" Word

Racism is the abusive "social construction and categorization of people based on perceived shared physical traits that result in the maintenance of a sociopolitical hierarchy." (APA, 2019) Race is defined by *Merriam-Webster Dictionary* as "any one of the groups that humans are often divided into based on physical traits regarded as common among people of shared ancestry." Although definitions of race historically included a biological/genetic basis, current scholarship is that race is a social and political construction with no basis in a coherent biological reality (APA Guidelines on Race & Ethnicity in Psychology, 2019).

The Black and White race construction in America continues to be widely accepted by society. This ideology is identified as social constructivism and impacts resource allocation. Merriam-Webster defines the resource as a "source of supply or support; an available means." Racism allows resources to be withheld because of race. Moreover, it is systemic and perpetual, and according to Robin DiAngelo, "Systemic racism is deep and highly adaptable." Education is a resource and an essential strategy to help maintain and advance the availability of community resources. Departed, renowned educational psychologist, Dr. Asa G. Hillard III described racism as, "a system that encompasses economic, political, social, and cultural structures, actions, and beliefs that institutionalize and perpetuate an unequal distribution of privileges, resources, and power between White people and people of color." He wrote, "This system is historic, normalized, taken for granted, deeply embedded, and works to the benefit of whites and to the disadvantage of people of color" (Hilliard, 1992).

Racism, Types, and Subtypes
from Derman-Sparks & Brunson Philips, 1997

Racism

- Belief in the superiority of one's own race and the inferiority of another race and the power to take individual or collective action against the racial group(s) deemed as inferior;

- Involves negative attitudes, feelings, and beliefs toward individuals based on their perceived racial group membership;

- Builds on belief of race as a biological concept, combines belief in racial superiority with a hierarchy of privilege.

Individual Racism

Individual behavior, the outcome of which reinforces a dominant/marginalized economic, cultural, sociological, and/or political paradigm, regardless of the individual's good intentions. An individual may act in a racist manner unintentionally.

Interpersonal Racism

Interpersonal racism occurs between individuals. Once private beliefs come into interaction with others, racism is now in the interpersonal realm. Examples include public expressions of racial prejudice, hate, bias, and bigotry between individuals.

Internalized Racism

This is loosely defined as the internalization by people of racist attitudes toward members of their own ethnic group, including themselves. This can include the belief in ethnic stereotypes relating to their own group. As proposed by Robin Nicole Johnson (*The Psychology of Racism*): "an individual's conscious and unconscious acceptance of a racial hierarchy in which Whites are consistently ranked above people of color."

Institutional Racism

An institutionalized system of economic, political, social, and cultural relations that ensures that one racial group has and maintains power and privilege over all others in all aspects of life. As such, racism is measured by its economic, cultural, sociological, and political *outcomes rather than by its intentions* (i.e., its effect on both racially and ethnically marginalized groups and racially and ethnically dominant groups) (Derman-Sparks & Philips, 1997). Institutional racism occurs within and between institutions. Institutional racism includes discriminatory treatment, unfair policies, and inequitable opportunities and impacts based on race produced and perpetuated by institutions (*e.g.,* schools, mass media). Individuals within institutions take on the power of the institution when they act in ways that advantage and disadvantage people based on race.

Systemic/Structural Racism

Structural racism is the normalization and legitimization of an array of dynamics–historical, cultural, institutional, and interpersonal—that routinely advantage Whites while producing cumulative and chronic adverse outcomes for people of color. It is a system of hierarchy and inequity, primarily characterized by White supremacy–the preferential treatment, privilege, and power for White people at the expense of Black, Latino, Asian, Pacific Islander, Native American, Arab, and other racially oppressed people in America.

Cultural Racism

Refers to representations, messages, and stories conveying the idea that behaviors and values associated with white people or "whiteness" are automatically "better" or more "normal" than those associated with other racially defined groups. Cultural racism shows up in advertising, movies, history books, definitions of patriotism, and in policies and laws.

Historical Racial Trauma

Trauma that is shared by a group rather than an individual and spans multiple generations who carry trauma-related symptoms without ever having been present for the past traumatizing event (i.e., slavery, forced removal of First Nations tribes from their land).

See the Bias

According to the Perception Institute, one way to combat our biases is to "identify responses rooted in stereotypes" (Perception.org, 2016). To transform the perception of Black boys, "Teachers who learn to appreciate their students as individuals will be less likely to default to stereotypes when viewing student behavior" (Perception Institute.com) Retired teacher Jane Elliot understood this principle and sought to disrupt stereotypes among her students. I recall seeing her story and demonstration played out on the Oprah Winfrey show in the 1980s, and again through her documentary during the pandemic in 2020, amid the racial justice uprising after the murder of George Floyd by police officers and an extremely discriminatory police system. Jane Elliot exposed her elementary school class to racism by dividing the class into two groups, blue eyes and brown eyes, and assigning privilege based on eye color. Her no-nonsense approach to exposing those of privilege (blue eyes) to the feelings of the oppressed (brown eyes) was groundbreaking in 1968 and still remains a powerful demonstration.

Previous reports have revealed that the persistent and substantial overrepresentation of Black students in special education has lasted for forty years (Ford and Russo, 2016) and that biased methods of identifying these students likely contributes to this outcome (Bean, 2013). Biased perception can keep pathways to meaningful engagement blocked and inform racist actions such as over-identification (and under- and mis-) in special education and discipline referrals. According to the Perception Institute, "Black boys' behaviors seen through the lens of implicit bias are interpreted far differently than the same behavior by a White boy", resulting in the disproportionality of referrals to school discipline in suspensions: 15% to 4.8% respectively (Perception.org).

Bias is a two-way street: Just as you have attitudes and beliefs of your students, they have attitudes and beliefs of you. Self-assessing your bias is a helpful first step. The Anti-Defamation League has an Anti-Bias Behavior self-assessment that is useful in helping to see bias in self.

Implicit and Explicit Bias

Implicit biases are:

> *Thoughts and feelings . . . we are unaware of (them) or mistaken about their nature. We have a bias when, rather than being neutral, we have a preference for (or aversion to) a person or group of people. Thus, we use the term "implicit bias" to describe attitudes toward people or*

> *associating stereotypes with them without our conscious knowledge. (Perception.org, 2022)*

Explicit biases are:

> *Attitudes and beliefs we have about a person or group on a conscious level. Much of the time, these biases and their expression arise as the direct result of a perceived threat. When people feel threatened, they are more likely to draw group boundaries to distinguish themselves from others. (Perception.org, 2022)*

Awareness of bias is an initial step toward change. Kirwan Institute Study for Race and Ethnicity at Ohio State University describes implicit bias as a "powerful cognitive mechanism" that can be mitigated through the practice of self-awareness. Developing an anti-bias mindset is a valuable professional and personal responsibility. There are several areas to see clearly to make changes in practice toward equity.

See Change in Bias

Professionals and organizations must reconcile with their past or current participation in the poverty and prison pipelines. Andratesha Fitzgerald, author of *Anti-Racism and Universal Design for Learning*, says that anti-racism is "A series of choices or decisions to uphold or dismantle racism." Organizations in the BSSN ecosystem have begun to make conscious decisions and to publicize those decisions. For example, in 2019, the American Psychological Association (APA) published ethnicity guidelines to encourage psychologists to consider how their backgrounds shape behavior. On January 18, 2021, The American Psychiatric Association (APA) issued a statement titled "APA's Apology to Black, Indigenous, and People of Color for Its Support of Structural Racism in Psychiatry" that states, "The APA apologizes for our contributions to the structural racism in our nation and pledges to enact corresponding anti-racist practices."

These are two examples that created awareness of new intentions and recognition of wrongdoing. However, they are not reconciliations. They do not come close to "settling any accounts" as Race Card Project Founder and Washington Post Columnist Michele Norris said in her opinion of 2020's events that triggered widespread reflection on race relations. She warned that "an epiphany is not reckoning" and that "We can't increase racial equity without eradicating white supremacy." Increasing racial equity, "requires a full reboot and a commitment to let go of the things to which people cling, consciously or subconsciously" (Washington Post, 2020).

See Changes in Assessment, Learning, and Teaching

Cultural Competence

Instructional strategies can be culturally competent and inclusive. However, not all culturally competent instructional strategies are anti-racist. Cultural competence is understanding and interacting effectively with people from other cultures. Anti-racism is defined as opposing racism and promoting racial tolerance. Anti-racist instructional strategies embed critical thinking, teach and model empathy, provide opportunities for giftedness, consider subcultures, and build character. Ally Author, Robin D'Angelo, says "Less racist" is not a fixed location based on good intentions, self-image, or past actions. It is continually strived for through ongoing and demonstrated practice and ultimately determined by people of color. Common behaviors, norms, artifacts, and values define subcultures or subsocieties. Experiences, expectations, and resources make each subculture different from the next. Teachers and staff can benefit underserved students by considering the ethnic groups from which students come and acknowledging the variation within ethnic groups.

Psychological Assessment Bias

Ascertaining the IQ of a BSSN is helpful in the obtainment of public and certain private resources, such as education programs and psychological services. IQ is not a predictor of character. It simply gives us information about the capacity to learn new information in the way that the early educators (e.g., Dewey) designed learning to be taught. Maria Montessori's model, however, was absent of such confined cognitive frameworks. Having observed lower socioeconomic class children in Italy for her education model, she crafted observation and concern for the whole child as the guiding methodology for facilitating learning in children.

Dr. Asa G. Hillard III, (also known as Nana Baffour Amankwatia) was an African American professor of educational psychology who studied indigenous ancient African history (ancient Egyptian), culture, education, and society. Dr. Hilliard was one of the first Black psychology pioneers in the 1960s who identified bias in psychological assessment. He saw that questions and answers were not reflective of Black students. According to his obituary, "He served as an expert witness in several landmark cases that have resulted in the elimination of admissions tests as the sole criterion for college admission and led to the revamping of achievement testing. He was a founding member of the National Black Child Development Institute."

Norms in assessment instruments used in identification and placement decisions determine what is "normal," and information outside of that region is considered below or above normal. In general, the norms for assessments used by psychologists and neuropsychologists are still largely not influenced by BSSNs. Non-Black experts design the majority of instruments, cohort samples are tested with White subjects, and the evaluators are still largely White, without cultural competencies. Dr. Joette James, a neuropsychologist, affirms that the concerns of racism in the assessment of the past, which Dr. Hilliard would have tackled, are normal now, of course, with some exceptions. She says they have "changed for the intelligence of tests with pretty equitable age and socioeconomic stats." She says the only issue might be if you are not from the US, an adult, or for the use of more specific tests which use a smaller sample size and demographic.

For cognitive neuroscience research, where achievement is normed on thousands of people, there needs to be more representation in research. Dr. James points out the need for "more students of color to participate" in the norming samples, but there are barriers. She says for example, "scanners should be more user friendly" because hair (Black crowns) might not fit into the scanners.

Dr. James says that performance expectations can be based on the assessor's perception. Black students with White assessors will underperform because of a lack of rapport and trust. Tests have limitations, and the human element permits making assumptions not grounded in research. She says "building" rapport and "cultural competence" are critical. Assessors need to be able to ask about racial trauma and family history effectively and report it sensitively. If not, the White neuropsychologist will continue to have a short interface with the clients and not get successful treatment. We agree that there is also the continued opportunity to call more Blacks to the counseling, psychology, and psychiatry professions.

Evidence-Based Interventions

Evidence-based interventions are strategies proven to work for students with similar characteristics. Evidence-Based Interventions or Practices (EBI/EBP) are classified for specific domains to address specific skills yet are not child-specific. To be considered evidence-based, an instrument or strategy must be demonstrated to be effective across multiple sets of students, peer-reviewed, and published in a reputable publication such as a professional journal. This is an expensive process and subject to inequity as completion of EBI validation is limited to those with the resources to collect data on their instrument or approach. Publishing will be limited unless peer reviewers who are well-respected in their domain (subject matter experts) can appreciate, validate practitioner data, and affirm solutions. Unless journals that make publishing decisions are owned by Blacks or become more inclusive, inequities will persist.

Sometimes, there are cultural strategies or instruments that the BSSN parent, therapist, and/or physician has seen as benefiting the specific BSSN. These child-specific strategies should be considered as part of classroom strategies. However, if the strategy is not formally recognized as an EBI, its validity is limited for/in an IEP, for example. Recognizing and revolutionizing EBI to embrace more BSSN-specific solutions and strategies will be necessary. The following are signs and strategies to apply:

Repetition-Based Learning

Repetition is an evidence-based strategy for many students across the neurodiversity spectrum. Repetition provides the structure and muscle memory needed for repeat tasks. When we accept Dr. Kunjufu's position on time spent, then for the majority of students with special needs, repetition should be applied with great fidelity in IEPs for BSSNs. Evidence-based repetition strategies include repeated reading and daily routines. Nowhere is an opportunity more on display for this repetition of skill than I have seen in quality kindergarten classrooms, pre-identification, and in LFI (learning for independence) programs where students are in a more restrictive environment toward a high school certificate, learning functional life skills rather than academic skills.

Children with difficulties with memory may require more repetition. Students impacted by trauma are likely to suffer from memory and/or executive function issues (National Child Traumatic Stress Network Schools Committee 2008), impacting their ability to follow routines. Trauma can have a detrimental impact on students' functioning in the school setting (Honsinger & Brown, 2019).

As an undergrad at Towson University, I read Dr. Jawanza Kunjufu's book: *Countering the Conspiracy to Destroy Black Boys* (1985). It is a small but powerful pamphlet-sized manuscript that describes the systemic factors surrounding Black boys and how they are excellent students until fourth grade, when the effects of the absence of the male role model manifests.

> **Parents of Black boys**, you must do everything in your power to ensure a positive trajectory by the end of age nine to help maintain the hope of having his mind and body home through high school!

> **Teachers of Black boys**, you must do everything you can to ensure a positive trajectory by the end of third grade to position him toward pro-social behavior and successful academic completion!

In 2021, I had the pleasure of participating in a webinar where Dr. Kunjufu was the keynote speaker. So much of what he described still rang true from 1993, when I had added his material to my armor for social justice through my campus leadership (for which I was awarded Outstanding Woman of the Year) at Towson University. He still describes the displaced appetite for poor role models and athletic achievement over academic attainment. No one can say it better, so I will quote him:

> *We have a million black boys who want to play in the NBA, only 400K will make it in high school, only 4K will play in college, and only 35 make it to the NBA, where only 7 will start." He says we ought to "Realize that the odds that what you do most, you will do best. If Black boys spent the same six hours a day on studies as opposed to basketball, they would become proficient in their studies.*
>
> *-Dr. Juwanza Kunjufu*

Effective Teacher Models

Since the '80s, renowned education change agent Dr. Juwanza Kunjufu, has highlighted the disheartening decline in Black teachers. According to NCES, 79% of teachers are White, 7% are Black, and 5% are Asian, American Indian/Alaska Native, and others. Of the 23% of teachers who are men, only 2% (1.9% actually) are Black men (NCES 2017–18). This is significant because of the high percentage of Black boys and girls without relatable and positive productive role models in school, where they spend upwards of eight hours a day. An affirming and effective teacher is to be accepted regardless of nationality or sex; we simply need Black men to be the dominant model in adolescence. Dr. Kunjufu, since the 1970s, has been describing that the absence of the male role model in the home, in school, and in faith leaves the developing fourth-grade boy to procure peer models, which as Dr. Kunjufu says, are "poor substitutes." A *positive* role model is a passive participant, whereas a *productive* role model recognizes his responsibility for actions and outcomes.

The Bureau of Labor Statistics defines special education teachers as those who work with students who have mental, emotional, and physical disabilities. The work of a special education teacher is incredibly demanding and, like other teachers, special education teachers often take their work home. The average age of Black special education teachers is 43 for men and 49 for women, whereas the shared average age is 42 for White men and women special education teachers (Zippia.com, 2023).The number of Black special education teachers, already at the disconcertingly low level of 11% in 2010 dropped even further to 9% by 2021, whereas 71% of special education teachers are White) (Zippia.com, 2023). Special education teachers in public schools are required to have a bachelor's degree and a state-issued certification or license, and earn a median salary of $65,910 (BLS.gov, 2023). Zippia reports that Black or African American special education teachers have the lowest average salary, at $47,733. Being overworked and underpaid is a proven formula for high turnover/low retention and Black special education teachers are no exception to the rule. Those who continue are to be admired and respected for their dedication to the students they serve.

My cousin, Todd, was a beloved Black male special education teacher in Ohio public schools. He had most recently served as an Intervention Specialist for his school district. Unfortunately, we lost him in 2022 during the devastating COVID-19 pandemic; he was 55. I recall his mother and sister saying that being a special education teacher exemplified his loving character. We need more Black male teachers like him for our BSSNs.

The academic pipeline does not bend toward teachers in general. Sharif El-Mekki, founder and CEO of the Center for Black Educator Development, is working toward change. For the Black community in Philadelphia, he seeks to enter 21,000 Black male students into the teaching pipeline. El-Mekki says that typical "Educators use the foundations provided by the Educator Prep programs. But most of these educator prep programs derive their understanding of the art and science of teaching and learning from White educational and behavioral theorists." Mainstream practices and theories of such contributors as Horace Mann, John Dewey, and Jean Piaget cannot address the needs of BSSNs or their lived experiences, mainly because they were not developed with such subjects in mind or in time. Instead, BSSN educational leaders ought to regard the practices of educational leaders such as Carter G. Woodson, Lucy Craft Laney, and Mary McLeod Bethune.

Building Our Network of Diversity (BOND) Project and Real Men Teach are two organizations in the DC-Maryland region working to increase the numbers and quality of Black male teachers. They see the value of Black male teacher in their perspective, compassion, intelligence, and high expectations. Moreover, they recognize the importance of reflective relationships between a Black boy and a Black man. Maryland State Board of Education (MSDE) produced a 16-point recommendation plan on Achieving Academic Equity and Excellence for Black Boys (AAEEBB) after convening a task force in the summer of 2020 to explore inequities and develop evidence-based strategies for improving educational experiences and outcomes for Black boys in Maryland.

Strengths-Based Learning

Acknowledging strengths is a strategy used throughout education. In special education, we look for students' patterns of strengths and weaknesses. In addition to academic, cognitive, and functional strengths, education teams might also incorporate strengths such as artisanry, athleticism, language, and core values, such as compassion and justice. Embedding the strengths of ethnicity into the strategy for BSSNs' success can also be within reach. Without a holistic approach to strengths, education programming fails to develop the whole child's academic acumen and functioning ability. According to Urban Education, three out of four gifted Black children never get identified. Homes and schools must be willing and able to educate BSSNs about their strengths and not deny them that affirmation.

Beyond, yet related to the strengths-based mindset is the Black Superiority mindset which flourished in the 1960s as culture revitalization and identity movements grew. Membership of mobilized groups began taking responsibility for the service and safety of the Black community. Themes such as Black Power, Righteousness, and Leadership were largely influenced by the multifaceted (in compassion and controversy), Huey Newton and the Black Panther Party, the Black Hebrew Israelite Culture Revitalizations, Malcolm X and the Nation of Islam, Pan-African groups, and many others. Huey Newton claimed that Blacks' superiority was evident in the ability "to endure the most vicious and savage period" and that "the strength of the genes" would carry on.

Interestingly, the Black Panther Party (BPP) was hailed for its support of the 1977 American Coalition of Citizens with Disabilities', 504 sit-ins inside the San Francisco Federal Building led by Ed Roberts, Judy

Heumann, Brad Lomax, and others. The goal of the sit-in was to persuade the government to enforce a long-ignored section of the Rehabilitation Act of 1973 for accessibility, education, and training rights. It lasted for almost a month, making it the most prolonged peaceful occupation of a federal building in the nation's history. Brad Lomax, a member of both groups, enlisted the BPP's help, bringing food and provisions. The Panthers brought hot meals and other provisions to the building daily, provided regular newsprint coverage of the sit-ins, and even paid for Lomax's trip to Washington to sign the rehabilitation act of 1973 alongside Judy Heuman, renowned disability justice advocate. "Brad was able to get the Black Panther Party to see that this was critical to the work that they were doing," said Judy Heumann, a demonstration leader. "He was the linchpin for that," said Corbett O'Toole, who took part in the demonstration. She wrote (in an unpublished memoir), "Without that food, the sit-in would have collapsed," and the 504 section of the Rehabilitation Act may not exist (New York Times, 2020).

Faith-Based Competencies

BSSNs are likely to be nurtured in homes with cultures inclusive of faith-based beliefs or spiritual values, and related practices are part of the culture they may bring to school. According to Pew Research Center, 74% of Black Americans believe in God as described in the Holy Bible. The 2019 report on *Faith Among Black Americans*, describes that "...when segregation was the law of the land, ...faith more broadly (than churches or mosques), was a source of hope and inspiration" (Pew Research, 2021).

Teacher preparation programs will want to address faith in context with spirituality, since the connection to spirituality and/or religion have consistently been linked to improvements in mental health and wellbeing (Gill, Barrio Minton & Myers, 2010). Spirituality is the "...developmental engine that propels the search for connectedness, meaning, purpose, and contribution. It is shaped both within and outside of religious traditions, beliefs, and practices" (Benson, et. al., 2003). Teachers with faith-based competencies will have powerful tools to broaden individual capacity and strengthen relationships in the learning community. Powerful tools include prayer or meditation to cope with reality, educational empathy to appreciate diversity among student peers, and focus (also referenced as mindfulness) to improve concentration (Jackson, 2017).

Spirituality in adult education could not have progressed without the power of voices such as bell hooks, who argued that it was time to "break mainstream cultural taboos that silence our passion for spiritual practice" (Hooks, 2000). Teacher preparation programs should help student-teachers recognize the distinction between spirituality and religion. Often used interchangeably, spirituality, religiosity, and faith are interrelated concepts (like ethics and morality) yet have different meanings. According to a Berkeley magazine, "A person often inherits religion, but makes the conscious choice to practice spirituality by seeking answers about the self, universe, and meaning of life" (Zakrzewski, 2013).

School activity exemptions are related factors to consider and support. Faith-based BSSN families may not be willing to participate in specific learning activities or attend enrichment classes or tutoring on certain days of the week, or may altogether be absent during weeklong observances. Also, school culture activities, uniforms for athletics or dance, or even curriculum materials may be averse to the faith convictions of some BSSN families.

Health-Conscious Learning

One of the best features I appreciate about preschool classrooms and Montessori classrooms, in particular, is how learners are allowed to eat when hungry. This practice recognizes that each learner is unique and may need or benefit from healthy snacks or drinks throughout the day, not only when the bell rings. Teachers always appreciate healthy snacks that promote learning in the classroom. Whether provided by parents or schools, high regard for snack and lunch quality should be evident in classrooms with BSSN. The CDC recommends that nutritional needs come from nutrient-dense foods and beverages, such as plain or fruit yogurts, low-sodium beans, fresh fruits, and water instead of soda (DietaryGuidelines.gov).

Group breaktime are another facet of "factory" education. BSSNs who benefit from exercise and rest periods ought to have regular access to calming spaces and opportunities for quiet. We will discover more ways to synchronize health and education in Chapter Five.

Behavior-Nurturing Strategies

Rather than *behavior management*, I use the term *behavior nurturing*. We want to nurture the behaviors we want to see, and the unproductive behaviors will then diminish. Parents and teachers reinforce expectations not by posting them or verbalizing them but by consistently demonstrating them. One evidence-based practice for this is teacher modeling and peer modeling, where the teacher or designated peer's practice is, "First I do, then you do," for example, in a primary classroom. Some schools will say it is commonplace and part of their teacher expectations; however, this is not always the case. For specific clients, I advocate that modeling be written in the IEP: "Given teacher (or adult) modeling…." (as part of the goal) and "peer modeling" (as an instructional support) are two common examples.

Parents often know best what behavior-nurturing practices will and will not work for their unique child. In the *P.A.R.E.N.T.S. Life Skills, Literacy and Leadership Framework for Social Change Workbook*, the (N) Nurturing competency as a life skill in the context of parenting is explained as:

> *Instinctively, parents will nurture what they know, are strong in, and have interests or abilities toward. Whatever you nurture or cultivate in a child, whether positive or negative, will, in most cases,*

> *grow within the child. Nurturing requires attention, and children benefit from parental affection. Affection is a stimulant for growth through methods such as touch and tone of voice. (Jackson, K. and Jackson, M., 2015)*

Not all students will respond to modeling; sometimes, what we ask them to do is beyond their present capability. According to Ross Green, his Collaborative and Proactive Solutions© model is based on the premise that "challenging behavior occurs when the demands and expectations being placed on a kid exceed the kid's capacity to respond adaptively…and that some kids are better equipped (i.e., have the skills) to handle certain demands and expectations." A complete Present Level of Performance (PLOP) will include the BSSN's current capacity to respond to certain expectations, among other performance measures. BSSN tend to have atypical development, co-occurrence of difference or disability, application of multiple interventions and supports, and changes in performance levels are subject to change. Therefore, the PLOP should be updated twice a year for certain BSSNs rather than IDEA's annual guideline. Parents must be included in conversations around behavior-nurturing strategies and consequences during the specialized education plan development.

Sex-Based Learning

Let us maintain sight of the value of single-sex classroom learning, where boys and girls are educated differently because of their differences. For example, girls tend to be more interested in fine motor than gross motor like boys, boys tend to want to showcase their egos more than girls, and girls tend to want to please the teacher and earn high marks more often than boys.

Dr. Kunjufu taught in his teacher preparation classes that, "…if labeled Special Ed in terms of Black children, 85% of the time it will be a black boy." He exclaimed that the real challenge is not the male students, but the persistent presence of the female teachers. He said that the school system has designed a classroom for female students. I remember an interview in 1988 where he recognized that Black and White boy students were having similar difficulties in the "female-run classroom." He said that if we know that boys generally have "higher energy" and "higher egos," then we have to offer "more movement" and "gross motor opportunities" in the classroom for example, yet, "many times we are not doing that."

In their book, *Helping Boys Succeed in School*, Rich Weinfeld and Terry Neu, language arts is highlighted as an area where boys struggle most. They say that "having all-boys classes would allow teachers to focus on boy-friendly strategies and to create an environment that would allow more boys to take risks." They also suggest the value of evidence-based strategies that benefit boys, such as including trusted adults and break opportunities. These evidence-based strategies could be included in BSSN IEPs. Before the pandemic, a colleague and I began to outline a new social-emotional inclusive school model for middle school boys of color. Our academy framework was based on giving boys the space, figuratively and literally, to strengthen their confidence, emotional resilience, and academic and community skills. I thought about that model frequently during and after the pandemic when all the learning pods were popping up as BSSN parents grasped for socially-emotionally safe alternatives for their boys.

Given what we know and what has been proven about the need for differentiation in learning for the unique needs of boys and girls, we can consider appropriate in-school strategies to support vulnerable and social-emotional differences.

An Evidence-Based classroom for BSSN should include the following:

- Highly nurturing female teachers for students through grade 3.
- Highly qualified teachers (HQT) for reading, math, and science instruction

- Highly qualified specialists (HQS) for speech, physical, and occupational therapies
- Black male teachers for boys in fourth grade and above.
- Outdoor or large spaces for movement and active learning for boys, in particular
- Learning stations with some space between them, for boys in particular
- A dress code, yet without uniforms
- Access to advanced academic work
- Restorative practices, to include parent and role model involvement
- Creation-rich curriculum with exploratory opportunities
- Skill building curriculum

Distance Learning

In March of 2020, the nation's exposure to the worldwide pandemic of COVID-19 required a national quarantine, closing schools and limiting community activities. After a few weeks, schools transitioned to distance learning to continue instruction for the remainder of the school year. Distance learning, also called Distance Education, is where instruction is not provided on-site. Instead, classes may be broadcast or conducted by mail or internet. Some districts carefully considered how to meet services remotely, and some still needed to. A Distance Learning Plan outlines the aspects of the IEP that can be accomplished in the distance education model. In other words, the distance learning plan identifies the aids or services from the student's IEP that can be delivered virtually. Aids, services, or accommodations in online learning that generally can be met are Graphic Organizers, Check for Understanding, and Speech-to-Text. Aids, services, or accommodations in online learning that generally cannot be met are: Preferential Seating, Physical

Therapy, and hand-over-hand: task guidance when the teacher's hand is over the BSSN's.

Digital Equity

While the COVID-19 pandemic advanced the applications of educational technologies, it also highlighted a gap in educational resources for underserved students. When almost all structured learning occurs online, acquiring skills in information technology and broadband access is a critical resource. The Digital Divide is the disparity in access to information technologies and digital services between different groups. For underserved students with special needs, acquiring information technology and skills amidst the pandemic was deeply concerning.

Moreover, inequities in digital services can present as inconsistent or limited broadband connections. For a child with an emotional disability, for example, frustrations with broadband can increase anxiety, decreasing the ability to attend to learning. These broadband gaps are particularly pronounced in Black and Hispanic households (Anderson, 2020). At the onset of the pandemic, only 67% of K–12 students had reliable access to computing devices; access levels were particularly low among low-income (52%), Black (58%), and Latino (61%) students. As schools shifted online, the digital divide may have worsened other inequities. Many students—particularly English Language Learners (ELL) and those with disabilities—rely on schools for occupational therapy, academic and social support, mental health care, and other services (Public Policy in California)

Learning Loss

Learning loss affected students across the world. In the U.S., the social-emotional impacts are still being felt by parents and teachers alike. Students are struggling with withdrawal and emotional regulation. For example, teachers report to me an uptick across general education in rudeness to teachers, calling out inappropriately, shutting down unexpectedly, inability to articulate their feelings and frustrations. BSSNs in general education can be supported through interventions and if unsuccessful, considering the process of identification for special education services described in Chapter 4.

In Indianapolis, the state anticipates it will take "another four years to merely catch up to 2019 proficiency levels, which were already too low to begin with" (The Mind Trust, 2022). 2021 was the first year students took a state assessment in Indiana. After the onset of the pandemic, students statewide saw an 8.5-point proficiency decrease from the 2019 ILEARN assessment, going from a 37.1% pass rate to 28.6%. In 2022, statewide student performance averages saw modest gains in ILEARN proficiency for grades 3-8: The statewide average pass rate improved by 1.7 percentage points to 30.2%. Statewide proficiency for Black students increased by 1.8 points to 9.9%. Statewide proficiency for Latino students improved by 1.7 points to 17.3%.

Access to learning enrichment after school and in the summer can help make up for learning loss. Black Students with special needs benefit from enrichment programming and the additional appropriate social opportunities. Removing barriers to access, such as transportation, cost, and unqualified teachers, can help BSSN experience successful enrichment. In addition, quality enrichment programs consider meals for families that may be food insecure.

Critical Thinking

Education has widely embraced critical thinking as an educational goal and norm for White students but not for Black students, based upon oppressive ideologies that Whites are superior intellectually to Blacks and, therefore, can naturally apply critical thought processes. However, critical thinking is not inherent to any race; it must be learned. John Dewey described critical thinking as reflective thinking. He defined it as "active, persistent and careful consideration of any belief or supposed form of knowledge in the light of the grounds that support it, and the further conclusions to which it tends" (Dewey 1910: 6; 1933: 9).

Teachers and staff can apply several strategies for critical thinking:

- Make group work productive by having participants clarify beliefs, values, or ideas.
- Encourage creativity and innovation from all students.
- Make critical thinking a habitual part of teaching and learning for all students.
- Incorporate independent and group problem-solving and expression of strategies.
- Encourage students to check their work.
- Share critical thinking activities with parents to use at home.

Empathy

Empathy is essential for cross-cultural relations, particularly relationships among dominant cultures and subcultures. Empathy, from the Greek, means having insight into another's reactions. Understanding why your students respond the way they do is empathy. You are empathetic if you can:

- See multiple perspectives;
- Avoid errors in judgment;
- Sense others' emotions; and
- Communicate emotions.

Empathy requires humility to keep in mind not only our own perspectives, but also those of others. Empathetic responses are acts of compassion and mercy. The Hebrew root word "rachum" means *womb*, where the most precious demand for compassion exists. It is imperative that we embrace the relationship of empathy, compassion, and mercy in the decision-making and resource allocation toward equity and justice for BSSNs.

Gifted Abilities

Black students with special needs can also be gifted. Gifted means having exceptionality in at least one academic area, artistry, and/or having a quantifiably above-average IQ. Academically gifted students require alternate instruction, classrooms, or placement for education enrichment. The education category for students with disabilities and giftedness is termed twice-exceptional, or 2E, because they need instructional and support plans specific to their disability that are also academically challenging. Thrice-exceptional, or 3E, is a newly coined expression to recognize BSSNs who are gifted. Exceptional BSSNs can be supported in school if teachers and staff:

- Invite culturally diverse guest speakers who can talk about their own experience with education and how they became successful.

- Engage parents and help them understand the entire evaluation and placement process; identifying giftedness can be a shared responsibility.

- Foster a sense of belonging in the advanced learner classroom through strategies such as conversation and pairing.

- Allow students to demonstrate their gifts in front of their peers.

Character Development

Each student will develop their own unique character. Instead of always telling students, ask what strategies and tools will help them make a connection to the curriculum. A good question is, "How would you like to demonstrate your learning?" Consider allowing submission of their answers in individual ways. Make sure that all instructional materials are accessible rather than generalizing fit. Ask BSSN, "How many words in the paragraph did you find difficult to read?" "Are you able to reach the supplies?" "Am I writing the examples too fast?" Include storytelling to build character. Encourage students to tell and listen to each other's stories. Provide tools for writing personal and fictitious stories related to their culture, gift, and/or disability. Using inquiry brings BSSN into the center of the decision-making process for their learning and growth in character.

Parent Engagement

Parents must be deeply invested in not becoming complicit. One way to do this is to ask questions. Regardless of the education environment type, parents ought to ask the following questions on behalf of their BSSN:

- Inquire about direct BSSN benefit: How will the classroom instruction and/or curriculum benefit my child?

- Inquire about your IEP or 504 plan implementation. How will my child's accommodations or supplementary aids and services be provided?

- Inquire about teacher preparation: What are the teacher's or specialist's experiences, skills, or credentials?

- Inquire about discipline methods: What are your behavior expectations, and how might you prepare for and respond to my child's challenging behaviors?

Parents are the first teachers for their children and their observations are essential in assessing developmental delays and academic abnormalities. However, even when parents of Black children bring their concerns to the attention of teachers or physicians, their concerns are often disregarded as unwarranted.

How to Achieve Identification Without Subjectivity?

The subjectivity of the process of identifying students with disabilities may impact racial disproportionality in that the cultural or racial bias of an educational team or its limited expertise can affect decision-making.

The more objective the process, the less chance that subjectivity and bias have room to influence outcomes, for example, in cases where the identification is made without psychological or other pertinent testing. We will explore this more in the next chapter.

Reflection Exercise:

1. Perform or complete a self-assessment of your Implicit Bias.
2. Review your results and choose one aspect of your bias for this reflection exercise.
3. Describe the context of your bias.
4. Answer: How has your bias caused any amount of emotional or physical harm?
5. Write an apology statement toward the person or persons. You do not have to send or share; the exercise is for your self-examination.

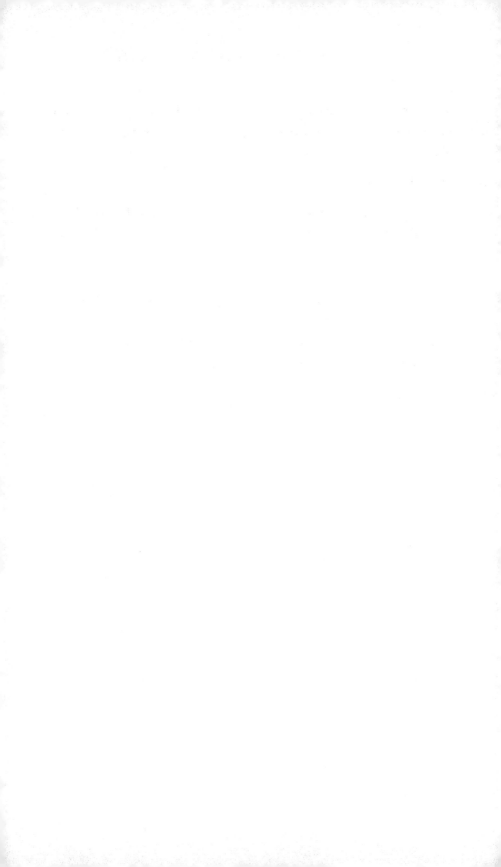

Chapter 3

See the Pipeline: Decisions, Discipline, and Disparities

CHAPTER INTRODUCTION

The continuous conduit of disenfranchised students, disciplinary activities, community crime, and incarceration is coined the school-to-prison pipeline. In this chapter, we examine the STPP (school-to-prison pipeline), hoping to turn off the special education inequity valve to the channel that has stolen, killed, and destroyed so many lives. The STPP is an interconnected system of poor health and nutrition, absence of role models, and widespread illiteracy (as tubes and cylinders) for moving frustrated, traumatized, anxious, and angry students (as harmful liquids and gasses) from school to prison (one place to another), without a fair return. Pipelines are designed to operate at high pressures and are often buried underground or submerged in water. Nearly 80 million juveniles and adults have been buried or submerged in this cycle of hopelessness.

James – A Fictional Case Study

The movie, *What to Do about James* is a 1970s film about a fictional character, James. The movie chronicled a few months in the life of a relatable yet fictional character, James Morrison. James was a boy BSSN, age 15, who had a developmental disability and who was loved by his mother, a single parent working two jobs and caring for an elder parent. The story tells of James's unconsciously incompetent law-breaking in the form of retail stealing, skipping school, and home burglary. His criminal activity is common among 5,000 other students arrested in the fictional city, and he is in one of only two special education classes at his school of 1,200 students.

Upon James's first arrest and questioning at the police station, he struggled to recall his personal identifying information. He could not identify his father and did not know how to reach his mother, who was not answering the phone at home. He did not understand his Miranda rights. He showed signs of emotional distress: He was in a daze, sweating, looking around in fear, crying, inability to answer questions directly or accurately, and not understanding what was happening. The police station staff said, "Calm down," and stated his charge—shoplifting—and tried to reassure him that they would find his parents.

Since they could not find his mother, he was detained in a juvenile detention center and had to go to juvenile court and be assigned an attorney. Since James was receiving special education services in school, his case was closed, and he was returned home. Subsequently, James appears in court a few times and the judge would rule his case as involved or not involved as an accomplice. During the movie, it was determined that James was a seventh-grade student with special needs. His mother described him as someone who was "slow" and "has trouble understanding." In addition, James was being bullied and groomed by a gang at school. His mother said the students are always "picking on him;" "I'm not sure what we can do."

James was remanded to a home detention program. A pupil personnel worker (PPW) tried to help by connecting James to a school counselor and searching for special schools that would take James. However, the school said that he could not go to a special school as that would be a duplication of services. At one point, the judge approved James for psychological evaluation. His mother expressed reluctance when the psychologist asked to leave him and James alone. After assessments and tests, it was determined that James was mildly mentally retarded (a label we no longer use), functioning at a seven or eight-year-old academic level, and had limitations in social judgment.

At one point, James was remanded to home detention, and the team explored the option of an adolescent intervention program. Throughout the movie, his mother emphasized that she had repeatedly asked for "help!" with James and that she does her best. She said, frustratedly, "I went to one place trying to get help, and they told me I make too much money, and I went to another, and they made it seem like something was wrong with me."

The PPW reported to the judge on his unsuccessful attempts to get the resources James needs at his school, or to find James a private school that fits within the funded criteria. James's attorney advocated that the courts, school system, and the community meet James's needs. James's mother admitted that it was hard to accept James's disability but that she was willing to do whatever it took so that James could get help. The judge voiced frustration in the absence of the school system's representation at any of James' court hearings. She realized that while the juvenile detention center was not the appropriate place for James, neither were the programs for the "severely intellectually disabled", and the "milder functioning" as she described, will not accept students with his acting out behaviors.

The movie ends with the judge saying, ***"I'm just not sure if in this city there is any help in the system for James."***

What Would We Do About James Now?

The dilemma of sufficient academic engagement for BSSNs boils down to leveraging advocacy, financial resources, and parent education. Without the advocacy from the PPW (and the judge), James's mother would not have explored school resources or private school options, James would not have been evaluated, and the judge would have ruled him involved in the justice system, which carries negative consequences for educational opportunities. The private schools considered were not behavior-matched for James, even though they served students with mild to moderate intellectual and emotional disabilities. In other words, the schools would not accept students with behaviors like James's. James's mother did not know the scope of his disability; she only knew that he was in a special program with learning disabilities. She knew she needed help with James, yet she also knew she did not appreciate having him evaluated without her presence.

When the movie was made in 1979, IDEA was fairly new (passed in 1975), so the language and processes in the movie were novel. Modern-day update: Private schools for students with disabilities are still very specific on the profiles of the students they will serve. School districts still need to refer more easily to those nonpublic options, especially if the programming and resources are provided within the public options. BSSN parents are still searching for help and are underinformed. Counselors are still limited in resources they can offer at school. PPWs, advocates, and attorneys are still brought into the picture too late. Judges interested in helping are still limited in referral options for BSSNs who are justice-involved.

Here are a few recommendations for professionals involved with BSSNs to mitigate justice involvement:

Suggestions for Juvenile Justice Staff like James's:

- Obtain training in de-escalation interventions and disability awareness, and learn how anxiety may present in BSSNs.
- Implement adolescent intervention programs, known today as restorative justice programs.

Suggestions for School Staff Like James's

- Teach James how to self-advocate in the case of a justice-involved situation.

- Connect families to PPW and counselors as soon as there is an indication of potential for a chronic situation or determination of educational disability.
- Administer appropriate evaluations to determine and update James's present levels of functioning and performance.

Suggestions for Moms Like James's

- Provide parent and alternate emergency contacts that the BSSN can memorize, or create an emergency information/contact card for the BSSN to carry with them.
- Seek resources of local advocacy groups, like the ARC in many cities, special needs PTA groups, and state-funded programs such as the Parents' Place of Maryland. Also seek out disability-specific parent groups with equity missions or committees focusing on students of color with disabilities, such as Dylsexia Advocation, Inc.

I interviewed Special Education Lawyer Michael Eig, a 40-year education law veteran, who played one of the attorneys for James in the movie. Regarding James's mother, who believed James was "slow," he said, "It has been a recent thing" that parents or professionals became engaged in special education. The tradition was that "you look after your own; families look after your own, and small towns look after their own." Even still, there are those who believe that "Black kids are not going to perform well." He says that "IDEA is the best special education in the world, even though we fight over it." He continues; "(fighting) is actually built into the law… it's raised the awareness" for Black parents in particular.

Attorney Eig said the judge's perspective on school placement limitations is still somewhat true. In "General Education, there is no individualization for students," and in special education, it is too prescriptive for some kids; "there's got to be something in between," he says.

Attorney Eig also shared that he has an idea for an IEP form redesign to satisfy the gap, promoting better parent and school engagement.

Attorney Eig says that as soon as defense attorneys see a case like the James scenario, the first step for them is to pull the education records. The records give the attorney something to rely on other than the parent or child's reports to determine what help they have been getting in school. Collaborating with an education consultant to offer insight into the records or serve as an expert witness is also helpful. He also says that interdisciplinary strategies and better tracking of data is necessary. As for James's mother, she was involved but overwhelmed by her obligations, lack of help, and the extent of his special needs. He says that the challenge and also the solution is to "harness the parental involvement" early on in the learning process because "by the time the parents get to us (attorneys), there is just anger and hurt," like James's mother felt.

As for the 1979 "What To Do About James," in 2022, Attorney Michael Eig said, "Programming is better," but "needs funding," and he said, "That title still works."

Nihcay – An Actual Case Example

Now, let us review a real case example, with the name changed to regard privacy.

Nihcay is a 13-year-old BSSN boy in a private school for students with disabilities like his. Nihcay's FSIQ (Full Scale Intelligence Quotient) is 101, spanning average to high average, which indicates that he has a high aptitude for discovery and retention of information. He also has a well-developed vocabulary and expressive language skills. However, in the speech and language area of pragmatics, there is evidence that he needs help with physical context, conversational skills, recognizing the audience, using purpose in conversations and communications, and recognizing nonverbal cues.

Nihcay benefits from a learning environment that can meet his grade-level skills and respond to his advances and interests in reading, writing, and math. He has difficulties and needs in the following: Social reciprocity and pragmatic language, fixated interests, reduced effect, limitations in sharing and imaginative play, worrying, task avoidance, and hypo/hyperactivity to sensory input and predictability.

In seventh grade, Nihcay was diagnosed with autism, anxiety, and ADHD. Given his disabilities, he needed accommodations, goals, and services to access his district's general education curriculum. Nihcay needed to learn to accurately integrate verbal and nonverbal communication (such as facial expressions and body language), initiate and maintain social interactions, apply coping and executive functioning skills through training, and given attention to tasks through reduced distractions.

Nihcay was born full-term and healthy. Nihcay met almost all his developmental milestones except for his vision. Early on, his mother and then eye doctor (after two visits), noticed that he had a slight strabismus, which eyeglasses have accommodated. His mother also noticed that Nihcay was having trouble with attention and early academics in kindergarten and beseeched the EMT (Education Management Team) to intervene. However, it took three years for a school team to identify Nihcay with an education disability and obtain special education services.

In early primary grades, Nihcay mostly met his grade-level writing, reading, and math benchmarks, although concerns regarding his attention-seeking work-avoidance and other behaviors resulting in peer conflict were noted by his classroom teachers. His parents requested a special education evaluation during his third-grade year, with results showing significant symptoms associated with ADHD, hyperactive-impulsive type. He also met conditions for a significant emotional condition. However, as the available data from his teachers were "not compelling for establishing an adverse educational impact as he continued performing on grade level with relative independence," he did not qualify to receive special education services at that time. In third grade, Nihcay was identified as a student with an emotional disability. He had difficulty making communicative connections with adults and peers, including inferring the intent and meaning of the conversation, often asking, "What do you mean by that?"

He would also misinterpret social contexts and remarks made by his teachers. Nihcay was assessed in the area of speech and language to evaluate his expressive and receptive language. Results indicated strengths in receptive vocabulary, sentence expression, and comprehension of orally presented information. Weaknesses included below-average scores in pragmatic language. However, it was determined that those scores were not "an accurate reflection of his pragmatic skill set," and he was not recommended for speech-language services.

His parents then homeschooled him for the first quarter of fourth grade due to his difficulties with transitions and other interfering behaviors. This homeschooling period helped Nihcay's parents to identify his strengths and needs better and try different environmental and educational strategies. They provided this information to the school team when he returned to school for the latter half of the school year.

His parents then submitted a second request for special education evaluation due to concerns about inflexibility, anxiety, and attention-seeking behaviors. Finally, at the start of the fifth-grade school year, Nihcay was found eligible. The psychological report supported that due to his "extremely high rate of anxiety, obsessive/compulsive behaviors, difficulty coping with stress, and an inordinate need for attention and interpersonal connectedness, as well as his disproportionate reactions to social situations," he qualified for special education services under the diagnosis of emotional disability.

Nihcay began receiving special education services in fifth grade in the areas of reading, math, and various behavior interventions at his home elementary school. The services carried over into middle school for sixth grade but were disrupted by the global pandemic and distance learning. Nihcay participated as best he could through the remote instruction's video conferencing tool. He would participate in only portions of the classes and spent time distracted by computer features unrelated to the assignment or instruction. Psychological services were only as productive as he was interested in talking or having his camera view in the "on" mode.

Another speech and language evaluation was performed. Additionally, other assessments, classroom observation, teacher reports, student portfolio, and Nihcay's educational history was reviewed. Based upon the comprehensive evaluation and review, it was determined that Nihcay's weaknesses in pragmatic language negatively impacted his educational performance in his ability to interact with peers and engage in higher-level classroom discussions appropriately. Nonetheless, his weakness in oral communication did not explain his broader difficulties with academic, social, or functional areas. Additional assessments were warranted to determine primary educational disability and the need for special education services.

Ultimately, through several school meetings at different levels, it was determined that Nihcay had a unique pattern of strengths and weaknesses that required more specialized interventions and services in a more restrictive learning setting. Since the district did not have such a setting, a private, diploma-track special education school was sought and provided to Nihcay at no cost to his parents. Nihcay is finally making progress, closing his multiyear academic gap, and looking forward to graduating high school with a diploma.

Debrief

Nihcay is an example of a BSSN who struggles in a typical school setting without HQCT (highly qualified and *compassionate* teachers), organized staff, appropriate interventions, and appropriate academic and social-emotional supports. Because his disability impacts his ability to socialize, without HQCTs BSSNs like Nihcay often wind up with failing grades and repetitive referrals to the principal's office. In addition, without effective interventions and strong parental involvement, BSSNs like Nihcay are frequently suspended and are vulnerable to the unproductive influences of peers or others in their community.

For example, given his language impact, a BSSN like Nihcay might ignore or respond rudely to teachers, staff, and peers. Additionally, he might not complete his assignments, be easily intrigued or distracted by peers, and ultimately begin antisocial behaviors in other settings. At school, the Nihcay-like BSSN might demonstrate such behavior at home and in his neighborhood also. For example, he might ignore his parents at home or yell at a sibling for minor infractions. In the neighborhood, he might use fighting to communicate or cope and disregard adults and authority in the community. Over time, a BSSN like Nihcay, without HQCT, well-functioning staff, appropriate interventions, and adequate parental engagement, would become disassociated with learning, disconnected from school through truancy and suspensions, and ultimately disenfranchised from the community.

However, the Nihcay-like BSSN could succeed with appropriate support through measurable goals and objectives, supplementary aids and services, classroom accommodations, evidence-based interventions, and related services such as speech and language, occupational therapy, and counseling for school-related problem-solving. With the appropriate support, he would be able to self-advocate for his needs and wants in a way that is effective and according to his ability, maintain conversations without communication breakdowns, and accept instruction from his trusted teachers and adults that he recognizes are not adversaries. His parents would be adequately trained on the nature of his disability, how it impacts him in his environment, and the kinds of interventions that would help. They would monitor his health and wellness and hold him accountable for practicing his coping and social skills. His parents would be active members of his education team, advocating for his support and services.

If the Nihcay-like BSSN does not receive appropriate interventions and support, the presentation of his disability would become unmanageable in the school setting. Students with special needs who do not receive appropriate services in school (nor home and community), have very poor outcomes like addiction, leading to crime and prison. Juvenile ADHD is a risk factor for addiction disorders and impaired social interactions in adults (Shankman et al., 2009). Unfortunately, for decades there has been a disparity between how Black and White students are identified and served in Special Education, and more despairingly, how they experience postsecondary opportunities—if they even make it that far.

Related Factors

Attendance

Irregular attendance can predict better than test scores do whether or not students will drop out before graduation. The web of challenges facing children living in poverty, such as housing or food instability, lack of access to quality health care, unreliable transportation, and parental mental health instability, make it harder to attend school regularly. Missed days, or absenteeism, can erode academic performance and social progress. According to Future Ed and AttendanceWorks, students who are chronically absent (those missing 10% of more of the school year in excused or unexcused absences), often struggle to read well by third grade, are more likely to drop out of high school, and less likely to persist in college (Jordan, 2019).

Even the best education setting is only effective if the child is present. If absenteeism is an issue, whether the setting is the appropriate placement should be considered as well. These absences are most 9prevalent in the first years of formal schooling (prekindergarten and kindergarten) and in high school, and they disproportionately affect students from low-income backgrounds (Lavigne, et al., 2021). I have worked with school-staffed PPWs (Pupil Personnel Workers) to help families create and troubleshoot bedtime and morning routines and connect to community resources to address chronic absenteeism.

BSSNs might also miss school out of concern for their safety. Threats from school bullies and community violence are valid concerns from students of all grades. According to a survey by US Centers for Disease Control, about 7% of high school students said they missed school in the past 30 days out of fear for their safety either at school or traveling there. Safety concerns are particularly a factor in disadvantaged communities in poverty.

Chronic Absenteeism

According to a report by the Department of Education, "Chronic Absenteeism in the Nation's Schools," when compared to White students, Black students are 40% more likely to lose three weeks of school or more. Hispanic students are 17%, and Native American and Pacific Islander students are over 50% more likely. Students with disabilities are 1.5 times more likely to be chronically absent than students without disabilities (Gottfried et al., 2019). Issues related to feelings of not belonging in general education, individual health problems, and school refusals (resistance to attending school) are reasons for chronic absenteeism. Attendance outcomes can be improved through greater awareness on the part of the school staff of the students' needs and issues, increased and improved teacher training, and greater regard to contexts, such as school climate. Additionally, improvements and integrations in health and care services, parent education, and family engagement will reduce chronic absenteeism.

School Disciplinary Actions

The wrong approach to school discipline can leave students feeling unsafe or unfairly punished, which can lead to chronic absenteeism. Some BSSNs (whether identified or not) might not recognize the value or feel a connection to teachers, students, or coursework. For BSSNs with emotional disabilities (ED) or autism, for example, these feelings of physical or emotional harm may or may not appear rational or warranted. However, they must be addressed and perhaps identified as school refusal—resistance to attending school, as a nature of the disability. See the parent testimony in Chapter 6 from a parent whose BSSN with ED struggled with school refusal.

Additionally, Black and Latinx students were often more likely to be targeted with metal detectors than White respondents, according to *Arrested Learning*, a 2021 report which surveyed youth on police and security at school. At metal detectors, 34% of Black respondents have had their belongings taken, compared to 14% of White respondents. 19% of Black respondents have been yelled at, compared to 8% of White respondents. 34% of Black respondents and 22% of Latinx respondents have been made to take off their shoes, versus 7% of White respondents (Hamaji & Terenzi, 2021).

According to the Office of Civil Rights Government Accountability Office 2018 report on discipline disparity, Black students accounted for 15.5 % of all public-school students. However, they represented about 39% of students suspended from school—an overrepresentation of 23 percentage points. Black boys and Black girls were represented by the same patterns—the only racial group for which both sexes were disproportionately disciplined. Black students with disabilities represented about 19% of all K-12 students with disabilities and accounted for nearly 36% of students with disabilities suspended from school— about seventeen percentage points above their representation among students with disabilities.

Prison, the End of the Pipeline

Discipline referrals to the school's administration lead to out-of-school suspensions. According to an executive summary by the Perception Institute: *Transforming Perception: Black Men and Boys*, "Black boys in particular appear to be referred for suspension more readily because their group membership leads them to be stereotyped as more threatening, disruptive, and uncooperative by teachers and school administration" (Perception.org). Suspending students has dangerous results, including missed time from class, which researchers have found can lead to more dangerous consequences, such as disenfranchisement, (losing the basic rights of life, liberty, and the pursuit of happiness afforded to citizens), and sliding into the school-to-prison pipeline (Cavanagh et al., 2014). When the school staff or parents cannot find the students during the day, then the police likely will. The school-to-prison (and to-deportation) pipeline refers to the policies and practices that punish, isolate, marginalize, and deny access to supportive learning for Black, Latinx, and Indigenous students.

> *A male student of color who is suspended is three times as likely to drop out of school by the 10th grade and is in turn three times as likely to end up incarcerated (Goertz, Pollack, & Rock, 1996). One little-known but chilling marker of this disproportionality is that, by the age of 15, roughly 2% of the black male American population is simply missing; these boys are neither in school nor in the criminal justice system. They are most likely alive, but they are utterly disenfranchised from society (Flynn, 2008). This is a fate suffered by no other demographic group in America.*
>
> -Perception Institute

According to the American Civil Liberties Union, 60% of people in local jails have some form of mental disability. When my husband and I taught parenting in prisons to men and women, at least 70% of our class participants received medication for a mental/emotional disability, had not finished high school, or were significantly illiterate. The percentage of adolescents with disabilities is 33% higher in correctional facilities than in public school special education. Additionally, Black students make up 50% of all students with disabilities in correctional facilities (Further et al., 2005).

The effectiveness of irresponsible discipline, including imposing punitive measures without understanding the consequences, may affect a student's outcome in their adult life" (Gregory & Weinstein, 2008). Incarceration and the death penalty for violent crimes are the real consequences of this understanding absence. Black youth are "almost five times as likely to be incarcerated as White peers", and "Twenty-two times more likely to get death if the victim is White" (The Sentencing Project at Equal Justice Institute, 2023) While the number of states which allow the death penalty is decreasing, in 2023, "nearly 80% of those executed lived with serious mental illness; brain injury, developmental brin damage, or an IQ in the intellectually disabled range" (Equal Justice USA, 2023) Dr. Joette James, a well-respected neuropsychologist, provides forensic evaluations for inmates on death row, to answer questions surrounding mental illness and developmental disabilities. She says that death row inmates have led extremely traumatic lives (including racial trauma), which typically yields them level 10 ACES (Adverse Childhood Experiences Scores), the highest.

Dr. James says that our focus should be on youth and prevention. Juveniles need proper evaluation, treatment for traumas, and therapeutic interventions to improve social relationships. If professionals understand that brains are not yet developed (and there could also be a disability to consider), they might be more likely to focus on restorative practices and programs. For example, states might adopt programs where offenders self-reflect and meet in groups with victims, complete probation, and have felonies wiped from their records. Dr. James says that the work is at the Juvenile justice system level; once they are in the adult system, they are lost.

Given America's cruel condition of police brutality, it is imperative that we keep BSSNs from interfacing with the justice system. As engagement in community crime increases as a result of school suspensions, expulsions, and detachment from learning is often a reality for BSSNs. Social scientists and public health scholars now widely acknowledge that police contact is a key vector of health inequality and is an important cause of early mortality for people of color (Edwards, Lee, and Esposito, 2019). The likelihood that police, rather than making a mental health response, will cite a BSSN with emotional disabilities in crisis as *"excited delirium"* or a BSSN with an intellectual disability with limited language as *"resisting arrest"* resulting disproportionately in the deaths of blacks, is a risk not worth taking. According to the article in the Virginia Law Review, entitled, *Excited Delirium and Police Use of Force:*

> *Of the 166 cases in which the race of the victim is available, 187 Black people make up almost half (43.3%) of the instances in which excited delirium is used to describe why a person died in police custody. When combined, Black and Latinx people constitute at least 56% of the deaths in custody in this sample attributed to excited delirium. This disparity reflects the disproportionate contact that police have with racial minorities as well as the persistent ways that race has framed excited delirium conversations since Charles Wetli and David Fishbain brought the concept into legal and forensic discourses. (Obasogie, 2021)*

Dominique Archibald is the mother of another by-police murder victim, Nathaniel Pickett. According to a 2021 NPR news story on fatal police shootings of unarmed Black people, where his father was interviewed, Nathanial was described as suffering from mental illness. However, the officer who killed him was cited as saying in court that it never occurred to him that Pickett could be mentally ill. NPR reported that Picket was diagnosed with mental illness in his first year at Hampton University in Virginia. Records show he had also received court mandated mental health treatment after a conviction for resisting a police officer and false impersonation. His mother, Dominique Archibald, said during the hearing of the International Commission of Inquiry, "We have more stringent rules of engagement and human rights requirements against the known enemy (foreign, wartime) than law enforcement has in the streets of America." Although Nathanial's family was awarded a settlement, his mother said, "You could never pay me for my child. Whatever comes is just a down payment on justice." (International Commission of Inquiry on Systemic Racist Police Violence Against People of African Descent in the United States, 2021)

As part of an effort to draw the United Nations' attention to police brutality, an alliance of leading human rights lawyers filed a comprehensive report against the U.S. for committing crimes against humanity. The report by the National Conference of Black Lawyers, International Association of Democratic Lawyers, and the National Lawyers Guild proclaimed that systemic racist police violence allowed law enforcement officers to kill and torture (chokeholds and violent restraints) African Americans with impunity. In 2019, Black and Indigenous people were three times more likely than White people to be fatally shot by police in the U.S. "Stunningly, for young men of color, police use of force is now among the leading causes of death" (Edwards, Lee, Esposito, 2019). Police employ a double standard; they see Black children as threatening and deserving of being killed. (International Commission of Inquiry on Systemic Racist Police Violence Against People of African Descent in the United States, 2021).

Chapter 4

Disconnect the School-to-Prison Pipeline: Align the School-to-Success Pathway

Different than a pipeline, a plumbline is used in construction and surveying to determine vertical alignment. It consists of a string with a weight attached to the end. A plumbline ensures that the walls, posts, and other vertical structures are straight and level. A primary difference between a pipeline and a plumbline is that a pipeline is used for transporting fluids in one direction, and a plumbline is used for measuring vertical alignment. The Recognition, Referral, Identification, Intervention, Placement, and Progression (RRIIPP) process outlined in the following pages is that necessary alignment. To enhance the application, reference the testimonies of Nihcay, and the fictional character, James, from the previous chapters.

RRIIPP is a descriptive framework for special education equity for BSSNs, based upon the IDEA law. I use the acronym RRIIPP to illustrate IDEA as a continuum with unbiased and effective impact to help disrupt the school-to-prison pipeline that misidentifies disabilities, improperly places students, lacks appropriate process, and overlooks potential, as seen in the 70% of inmates who cannot read beyond the fourth-grade level.

RRIIPP

- **R**ecognition of disability/delay by parents
- **R**eferral by physicians and specialists

- **I**ntervention by teachers and specialists
- **I**dentification by teachers and staff
- **P**lacement by education teams
- **P**rogression by teachers and parents

Disproportionate identification generally refers to group differences in the rate at which one group is assigned to a category at a higher or lower rate than that of students from other groups (Morgan, 2020). Conversely, proportionate representation occurs when students of one race/ethnicity are assigned to a category at the same rate as students from other groups are. Overrepresentation takes place when a group is represented at a higher rate in a category than the rate at which other populations are represented, and underrepresentation occurs when a group is represented at a lower rate. (Morgan, 2020) One of the methods for determining if a given group is overrepresented is the composition index. This method involves comparing the ratio of pupils from a particular demographic group identified for special education with the ratio of pupils of the same group within all of the student population (Counts, Katsiyannis, & Whitford, 2018).

This **RRIIPP** process is significant in correcting the school-to-prison pipeline which has touchpoints across multiple settings and sectors. Given that the initiation for recognition of a child's special needs and consent for referral primarily lies with the parents, home is the first line of defense. Decades of data comparisons show that the ethnic profiles of populations most affected by special education inequity are Black, Indigenous (Native Mexican and Native American), and Latino, with Asian and White as least affected. The disparity, as described by the data throughout this text, shows disproportionality in determinations and outcomes related to graduation, employment, deportation, incarceration, and death by suicide and violence. Multiple research studies also demonstrate that a child's race and ethnicity are significantly related to the probability that he or she will be inappropriately identified as disabled (National Research Council, 2002; Losen & Orfield, 2002). Disproportionality is due to "institutional racism, stereotypes, cultural incompetence, racial bias, and inequitable discipline policies" (Lehr et al., 2006).

Throughout the entire **RRIIPP** process, parents should be active participants and supported and integrated as essential team members at every meeting. Where applicable, the BSSN should participate in IEP or 504 plan meetings to practice self-advocacy.

RRIIPP: Recognition

Observation and validation of difference, disability, or gift by parents and physicians of possible specialized need for intervention

For many parents of BSSNs, child rearing, coupled with the investigatory task of recognizing developmental delays, is quite the challenge. BSSN parents face an inordinate amount of stress, bias, traumas, racial microaggressions, and, in many cases, financial constraints. These stressors can create discomfort, feelings of anxiousness, disengagement, and imbalances in work and home life. Many BSSN parents do not always have the benefits leisure time to observe their child. Abnormal child development and subtle differences in behavior may be overlooked when parents are disengaged, inattentive, uninformed, and under-resourced.

Recognition can be even more difficult for some BSSN parents who are single fathers or single mothers. Research shows that children in single parent households score below children in two-parent households, on average, on measures of educational achievement (Amato et al., 2015). According to the 2021 census, 64% of Black children, 50% of Native American children, 24% of White children, and 15% of Asian children are raised in single parent households. The rise in child poverty since the 1960s associated with single parenthood (largely facilitated by the AFDC: Aid to Families with Dependent Children and its protected entitlements effects) has negatively affected children's educational outcomes (Amato et al., 2015). The Russell Sage Foundation reported that the two-parent Black household has continued its disturbing downward spiral, with two-parent households plummeting from 67% in the 1960s to 37.7% by the 1990s (Tucker, et al., 1995). Moreover, the 1980's mass incarceration epidemic affects the Black father more than any other to this day.

Misunderstandings of functional and personality-specific behaviors of BSSNs are problematic among parents and teachers. Age-appropriate behavior, communication, and abilities can vary among children, especially ethnic children, given cultural and environmental differences and expectations; generalizations by childcare providers can be dangerous. Specialized parent education in developmental milestones and behavior, observation skills, and communication supports are needed to help parents better recognize and communicate about their child with care providers and physicians. As parents develop recognition and communication skills, childcare providers and physicians must also address their range of ignorance and biases.

BSSN parents also struggle with recognizing and then revealing observed behaviors that lead to labels like ADHD, for example. They often feel like it is a permanent declaration of inability, or that they are going against their belief in supernatural healing power. When deliberating on whether to accept or disclose observations, BSSN parents might consider the following:

1. Acknowledging observed behaviors does not have to lead to a diagnosis.
2. Receiving treatment for a medical condition is not by itself a sin or lack of belief.
3. There are many ways to address ADHD characteristics and behaviors.
4. Girls and boys can present differently.

It is imperative that parents work to obtain a comprehensive treatment plan for their child. It is extremely dangerous for a BSSN struggling with impulsivity to be without a comprehensive treatment plan as BSSNs do not get the benefit of the doubt in this society. Impulsive acts by Black students are not met with the same grace as those of White students with similar conditions.

BSSN parents frequently struggle to have their child's condition or behavior validated by physicians and specialists. Black parents must often see multiple specialists before their children finally receive a diagnosis (Constantino et al., 2020). Black parents, on average, made three times more visits to doctors to obtain an autism spectrum disorder diagnosis than their White counterparts (Mandell et al., 2009).

Results for recognition or diagnosis vary by region and can depend on family access to insurance and disability type. Dr. John Constantino, Director of the Developmental and Intellectual Disabilities Research Center at Washington University in St. Louis, examined the experiences of over 500 Black families affected by autism spectrum disorder in the United States and found a three-year delay in diagnosis. BSSN parents first noted concerns about their child's development around 23 months of age, told a professional six months later, and did not receive an autism diagnosis until their child was over five years old (Constantino et al., 2020). Moreover, Dr. Constantino's research supported the CDC's findings of Black children's comorbidity rate of autism and intellectual disability at 47%, nearly double that of White children (CDC, 2020). Black children with intellectual disabilities receive an autism diagnosis an average of six months later than comparable White children (Dryden, 2020).

Since parents are the expert early observers, parents should (a) balance their discoveries with developmental milestones, family history, and environmental contexts, and (b) be assertive and relentless for answers and access whenever they perceive a delay or disability. Unfortunately, however, often Black parents do not have the same quality or quantity of resources to win the battles against physicians, specialists, and educators who may be restrained by their unrecognized bias. Medical and educational professionals have the responsibility of ensuring that brown-skinned children are equitably valued for their potential and have the right to receive accurate identification and appropriate intervention.

The integration of health equity principles into practice is vital to address the structural and systemic inequities that drive disparities among children of color and minoritized populations in general (Wright et al., 2022). The racial and social biases of physicians can be explicit or implicit. Biases about pain tolerance and false narratives about the promiscuous nature of Black women were generated by owners during slavery to justify their overwork, sexual abuse, and rape of enslaved workers. According to the Jim Crow Museum of Racist Imagery, these false narratives continued into modern gynecology, which has its origins in research and experimental treatment *without anesthesia* on enslaved Black women. (jimcrowmuseum.ferris.edu, 2024)

The pervasive social narratives about pain tolerance are perpetuated by the sciences. For example, a 2016 NIH study of White medical students and residents demonstrated that endorsement of false beliefs about how Black people experience pain was associated with lower pain score assessments and inaccurate treatment recommendations for Black patients compared to White patients in mock clinical scenarios.

While race policies in pediatrics are being addressed, implicit bias is a harder and more pervasive problem. In 2009, NIH published a study on physicians' implicit and explicit attitudes about race. It measured implicit and explicit attitudes about race using the Race Attitude Implicit Association Test (IAT) for over 400K medical doctors and other physicians/physician-related professionals. It showed an implicit preference for White Americans relative to Black Americans. Participants were asked to link "images of black and white faces with pleasant and unpleasant words under intense time constraints—they tend to associate white faces and pleasant words (and vice versa) more easily than black faces and pleasant words (and vice versa)." The strength of implicit bias exceeded self-report among all test takers except African American MDs. African American MDs, on average, did not show an implicit preference for either Blacks or Whites, and women showed less implicit bias than men (NIH, 2009).

Proper Recognition leads to more accurate Referrals to specialists, assessors, and recommendations.

R*R*IIPP: *Referral*

Notification of observations and evidence to Physician and/or School with parental consent by physician and teachers to specialist or school admin

Child Find is a part of the IDEA which requires that all school districts identify, locate and evaluate all children, with disabilities, regardless of the severity of their disabilities. Each Local Education Agency (LEA) must locate, identify, and evaluate all children with disabilities who are enrolled by their parents in private, including religious, elementary, and secondary schools located in the LEA. (USDE, OSEP) Parents, physicians, and teachers are the primary referral sources of students with disabilities to schools' Child Find services. According to a 2019 Government Accountability Office report, "Among families of students with disabilities, those with lower incomes and who have children of color are less likely than their affluent and white counterparts to access their legal rights under IDEA" (GAO, 2019). Weinfeld Education Group Director, Rich Weinfeld, says that while his group serves mostly White and affluent parents with special education advocacy, he has implemented several services to reach families of color.

An accurate diagnosis of a developmental disability is critical and almost as challenging to obtain. There is a complexity of overlap as ADHD, learning disabilities, and developmental/cognitive disability sync 32% of the time. U.S. Centers for Disease Control and Prevention show that 22% of White children with autism also have an intellectual disability, but among Black children, the rate of intellectual disability in those with autism is over 44% (Dryden, 2020).

One advocate colleague had this to say about the content of this book,

> *I'm really hoping you'll emphasize the idea of referring for consideration of all possible disabilities. For example, if the child is misbehaving, might there be an underlying LD (learning disability) or OHI (other health impairment)? Their (the physician's) words to the parents and any letter they write should reflect that.*

This graphic outlines ten steps physicians and parents together can follow to support the referral process. Disproportionality is affected by the underdiagnosis of educational disabilities. According to the Journal of Child Psychology, students who exhibit ADHD symptoms such as hyperactivity yet are not clinically diagnosed as having ADHD (subthreshold students) are not receiving services. Psychologists Dr. Russel Barkley and Dr. Umar Johnson have distinct views on the issue of ADHD diagnosis. Despite the rationales for diagnosis, parent apprehension to assess is pervasive and understood, given a lack of holistic treatment offerings (in school and out) and/or various stigmas that we will explore in a later chapter. These subthreshold students do not receive appropriate resources in school but receive significant resources by way of corrections costs per inmate. In other words, the school-to-prison pipeline is fueled by subthreshold syndrome disorders. Subthreshold conditions may represent good targets for preventive interventions (Shankman et al., 2009).

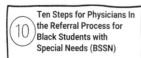

Ten Steps for Physicians In the Referral Process for Black Students with Special Needs (BSSN)

1. Discuss
2. Screen
3. Observe
4. Evaluate
5. Diagnose
6. Refer (Specialist)
7. Refer (School Team)
8. Recommend
9. Report
10. Discuss

Teachers are essential parts of the Individuals with Disabilities Education Act which includes the Child Find mandate. This obligation to identify all children who may need special education services exists even if the school is not providing special education services to the child (Wrightslaw.com, 2022). Teacher referral is a strong predictor of eligibility for special services. When Teachers refer to academic problems, 73-90% of students are found eligible, which is all the more reason to be very considerate and unbiased (Harry & Klingner, 2014).

While decisions are expected to be student-specific, studies have shown that physicians and teachers have racial bias. Students with an educational disability can be referred to the special education eligibility process by parents/guardians, physicians/therapists, or teachers/staff. Teacher referral is the strongest predictor of eligibility for special services. The existence of teacher bias is unfortunate, for teachers have such a powerful voice when it comes to eligibility determination. The practice of teacher bias in the special education process leads to misdiagnosis and inappropriate services.

RR*I*IPP-Intervention:

Services, supports, and therapies to address low performances and developmental delays by parents, providers, and educators through Referral to resources, programs, data, and evidence-based instructional tools.

One of the principles I learned in Facilitative Leadership training was that "An ounce of prevention beats a pound of intervention." In other words, it is always better to prevent a gap from widening or a delay from furthering. When prevention is not applicable (or is not effective), then interventions are needed; the earlier, the better. IDEA's Part C services provide early intervention for infants and toddlers (birth to age three) with disabilities. Services include comprehensive evaluations, an Individualized Family Service Plan (IFSP), and related services and therapies to be provided in the home or other natural environment.

However, given errors in recognition and referral, Black infants and toddlers with special needs often miss out on the opportunity to engage and benefit from early therapies. Using Dr. Constantino's study as an example, most of the 584 Black children with autism were diagnosed outside of the window to have received early intervention through IDEA's Part C services. Part C is supported by the "urgent and substantial need… to recognize the significant brain development that occurs during a child's first three years of life." More on the recommendation to prioritize early intervention in a later chapter.

The disparities continue beyond diagnosis in access to intervention services (Constantino et al., 2020). Limited access to specialized programs, services, and advocacy demonstrates decreased access to early intervention (part C) services among Black than White. According to research from the National Institutes of Health, "Black children are five times less likely to receive early intervention services than White children" and more likely to need it (Feinberg et al., 2011). The long-term impact of this disparity is despair, evident in American prisons and funeral homes.

Response to Interventions for BSSN

In secondary education, Interventions are practices or programs that, when implemented with fidelity, produce results and improve outcomes for students. Teachers apply targeted and intensive interventions depending on student needs, usually identified in an IEP. A Response to Intervention (RTI) Pyramid illustrates the progression of intervention each tier provides, whether evidence-based individual or group instruction. Black Students with Special Needs benefit from interventions that are targeted to their unique learning profile, with the consideration of cultural context.

Collecting performance data throughout the general and special education process is essential. Teachers, staff, and advocates use running records, formal and informal assessments, evaluations, and records of observable behaviors. Once an intervention is assigned to close a gap, monitoring is critical. Record-keeping strategies and intervention progress are essential to ascertain if the intervention was successful.

When RTI is applied effectively, it can eliminate cultural bias. As BSSNs progress through tiers of interventions, teachers should consider the following:

- Asking the Multi-disciplinary Team for additional resources, particularly if at or approaching Tier III.

- Avoiding *deficit thinking*, a racial bias where a student's performance is attributed to negative inferences such as "she is just not motivated" instead of evaluating school practice or process as a cause of low performance.

- Scheduling time for regular screenings and progress monitoring.

Once interventions have been explored, applied, and evaluated, appropriate identification can be made.

*RRI*I*PP: Identification*

by evaluations, data, parents, education teams, and experts to determine special education eligibility and gifted services

According to IDEA, in the 2020-21 school year 7.2 million students aged three to 21 receive services and are identified with educational disabilities. 17% of those students were identified as Black/African American. The SLD (specific learning disability) is the largest disability category, and on the opposite end, less than .5% of students are in the category of those with orthopedic impairment, visual impairment, traumatic brain injury, and deaf-blindness. According to the Brookings Institute, "...*aggregate* disability rates—with no adjustments for family income or other student characteristics—are higher for students who are Black (1.4 times) or Native American (1.7), and lower for Whites (0.9) and Asians (0.5), with Hispanic students about as likely to be identified as the rest of the population" (Gordon, 2017). Under the Child Find mandate, schools are required to locate, identify and evaluate all children with disabilities from birth through age 21. For example, BSSNs who have chronic or acute health impairments such as asthma, sickle cell anemia, lead poisoning, epilepsy, or diabetes might have limitations that impact their access to education.

The Child Find mandate applies to all children who reside within a state, including children who attend private schools and public schools, highly mobile children, migrant children, homeless children, and children who are wards of the state (20 U.S.C. 1412(a)(3)). This includes all children who are suspected of having a disability, including children who receive passing grades and are "advancing from grade to grade" (34 C.F.R. § 300.111(c)). The law does not require children to be "labeled" or classified by their disability (20 U.S.C. 1412(a)(3)(B); 34 C.F.R. § 300.111(d)).

Learning Disability

Black students are 40% more likely than their peers to be identified as having educational disabilities. Cognitive psychologist and author Diane McGuinness cites research showing that for many students, instead of attentional difficulty causing learning failure, failure to learn causes frustration, disinterest, and inattention (McGuinness, 1999).

Using ESSA's regulations can be a key strategy for identification (or determination) a disability in reading, for example:

"In making a determination of eligibility under paragraph (4)(A), a child shall not be determined to be a child with a disability if the determinant factor for such determination is—

(A) lack of appropriate instruction in reading, including in the essential components of reading instruction (as defined in section 1208(3) of the Elementary and Secondary Education Act of 1965)

(B) lack of instruction in math; or

(C) limited English proficiency." (20 U.S.C. 1414(b)(5)(A))

However, ESSA maintains the reference to the term *"essential components of reading instruction,"* which is defined as:

. . .explicit and systematic instruction in:

(A) phonemic awareness

(B) phonics

(C) vocabulary development

(D) reading fluency, including oral reading skills

(E) reading comprehension strategies

Maintaining this reference is essential since eligibility for special education services—particularly for a learning disability such as dyslexia—should not occur until and unless the student has received reading instruction that incorporates all of the essential components of reading instruction. Too often, students are found eligible due to poor reading instruction rather than the presence of a learning disability.

Educational Disability

Between the ages of six to eleven, on being identified with a disability, Black students have a risk ratio of 1.4, (White students have a .9) and are twice as likely to be identified as having emotional disturbances and intellectual disabilities as their peers." (GAO, 2019). Assessments, typically in the form of questionnaires, academic tasks, and problem-solving activities are used to determine disability. You might recall the 1974 Good Times episode, "The IQ test" (Season 2, Episode 7), where Michael performed among the school's lowest on the biased I.Q. (Intelligence Quotient) aptitude test because he refused to complete the test. The depiction was based on actual concerns of the time that as Michael put it, the test "was given by white people, made up by white people, and even graded by white people." Neuropsychologist Dr. Joette James says that racial bias in assessment, while not as pervasive, can still be a factor in pediatric psychological and neurological assessment. A source of bias for evaluators includes family belief systems about illness and disability, which impact a child's motivation and effort (James & Jackson, 2021). Unfortunately, due to systemic racism, observed discrepancies may be accounted for by psychosocial factors such as low socioeconomic status, unsafe living conditions, absent family members, poor parental education and occupational status (James & Jackson, 2021).

Intellectual Disability

Disorders usually present at birth (perhaps through genetics) uniquely affect the trajectory of the individual's physical, intellectual, and/or emotional development, with varied degrees of affect on multiple body parts or systems. Down syndrome is a great example of an intellectual disability. Down syndrome is a genetic disorder caused when abnormal cell division results in an extra full or partial copy of chromosome 21. This extra genetic material causes the developmental changes and physical features of Down syndrome (Mayo Clinic). Down syndrome rates increased over time among individuals who identify as Black, Hispanic, but not among white or Asian individuals (AJOG, 2022). Racial disparity in risk factors includes treatment for congenital heart conditions like atrial septal defect and the insurance or funding for proper care.

Developmental Disability

Not uncommon for students with special needs, BSSNs may have more than one disability or condition impacting their learning and function. Retired developmental pediatrician, Dr. Daniel Shapiro, says that screening for overlap in developmental disorders should be normalized. In other words, if we identify one developmental disability such as autism, we mind as well screen for ADHD, for example. Issues surrounding self-regulation is a broad theme across developmental disabilities. For example, BSSNs with autism can hyper-focus, and BSSN with ADHD can be easily distracted. Depending on the BSSN and conditions, these behaviors can co-occur.

Developmental differences are a combination of naturally developing and nurture-rearing factors. *Developmental disabilities* are a group of conditions due to physical, learning, language, or behavioral impairments. These conditions begin during the developmental period, may impact day-to-day functioning, and usually last throughout a lifetime (CDC), requiring specialized healthcare and educational interventions.

Not everyone with a developmental difference is impaired. However, everyone with a developmental disability has a developmental difference. According to the CDC, approximately one in six children or 17% of children ages three to 17 have at least one developmental disability, with 6.7% having two.

The unique needs of the BSSN, including performances in the classroom and results of evaluations, are examples of evidence to use when making disability identification or determinations. It is notable, however, according to research in *Unmeasured Confounding and Racial or Ethnic Disparities*, that Black students are less likely overall to be identified as having a disability. Yet when identified, they were 2.22 times higher with intellectual disabilities and 2.08 times higher with emotional disturbance than White students in the same 6 to 21 age range (Morgan, 2013).

See the end of the chapter and appendix for a full listing of IDEA disability categories.

*RRII**Pp**: Placement*

Matching BSSN with programs and schools, with input from parents, education teams, and experts to receive services, accommodations, and evidence-based interventions

Depending on their individual needs, the BSSN may need to be in the least restrictive environment inside of general education classes at the home school. This placement allows the BSSN to learn from and socialize with typically developing students as models and for the services, supports, and education accommodations for medical conditions, gifts, and disabilities provided in the general education setting. A self-contained classroom with only other students with disabilities is an example of a more restrictive environment. Depending on the disability and needs of the BSSN, placement in a specific program (including a nonpublic) to meet his/her needs may be war-ranted. Between 2007 and 2011, the percentage of students with disabilities (SWD) educated in SWD-majority classrooms declined nine percentage points while the percentage educated in GEN-majority classrooms increased correspondingly (Stiefel et al., 2018).

Twice-exceptional students receiving GT/LD services demonstrate superior cognitive ability in at least one area and typically have production problems, particularly in the area of written expression. GT/LD services provide students with specialized instruction, adaptations, and accommodations that facilitate appropriate access to rigorous instruction in the least restrictive environment, which may include placement in Honors or Advanced Placement classes and access to the acceleration and enrichment components.

To avoid missed opportunities to recommend appropriate placement of BSSNs, schools should inform parents of these opportunities. BSSN parents should be involved in placement decisions and in the annual IEP meeting to determine if the placement is still warranted. BSSN parents can also visit the programs before enrolling. Here are a few questions BSSN parents might ask:

- How many other students are in the class, and what are their special needs?
- What is the student-to-adult ratio?
- What resources does the program provide?
- What are the staff titles and qualifications?
- What do other parents have to say about their experience?

RRIIP*P*: *Progression*

Education teams use evidence-based and appropriate measures of progress

Under ESSA, states must administer an annual, summative assessment to capture student achievement in mathematics, English/language arts, and science for use in accountability plans and to meet transparency reporting requirements. The widespread cancellation of testing in the Spring of 2021 was the first time a nationwide assessment waiver had been issued since the passage of the landmark education law.

The 2017. Federal legislation resulting from, *Endrew F. v. Douglas County School District, Colorado Department of Education* regarded academic progress. The preexisting IDEA guidance that the IEP be "reasonably calculated to enable [him] to make some progress," to emphasizing making appropriate progress. The order cited, "When all is said and done, a student offered an educational program providing 'merely more than *de minimis*' progress from year to year can hardly be said to have been offered an education at all."

One component of a FAPE is "special education," defined as "specially designed instruction . . . to meet the unique needs of a child with a disability" §§1401(9), (29).

> *A child's IEP need not aim for grade-level advancement if that is not a reasonable prospect. But that child's educational program must be appropriately ambitious in light of his circumstances, just as advancement from grade to grade is appropriately ambitious for most children in the regular classroom. The goals may differ, but every child should have the chance to meet challenging objectives. Justice Roberts, SCOTUS*

The IEP is the instrument by which performance data is gathered, measured, and reported. A purpose of an IEP is to track whether meaningful progress is being made. Measurable goals are drafted and finalized with input from the team, including the parent(s). Parent input can be a written narrative or presented verbally at an IEP meeting. Once the goals are finalized, the progress toward those goals is to be monitored, tracked, and reported upon. At least every nine weeks, goals are measured, and progress reports on goals are provided to the parent to review and discuss as needed. The goals are set once a year, to be achieved within that year, making sufficient progress each quarter. Attorney Eig says that "measuring and monitoring" is the key and where district funding should be allocated.

When goals are met, the team meets again to provide performance updates and set new goals if applicable When goals are not met from quarter to quarter, or from the beginning of the school year to the end, or even year over year, the IEP team needs to meet and discuss. Validating sufficient progress might include evaluating work samples or data records, which teachers should maintain and parents should view. When BSSN parents need clarification, the case manager (if IEP) or counselor (if 504) ought to provide or facilitate the provision of that clarification.

BSSN parents might notice, for example, a disparity between instructional level and grade-level performance. For example, the instructional level is grade eight, but the student's ability to perform is at the fourth-grade level. For several reasons, BSSNs may not always demonstrate competency in standardized assessments or class tests. Below are some of the most likely reasons BSSN may not perform well on tests/assessments. BSSNs:

- May need to *demonstrate their knowledge differently* through alternative demonstrations, assessments, or expressions.

- May have *test anxiety*, an extreme, debilitating psychological experience before/about testing).

- May have *task avoidance, a* symptom of a condition displayed as averting unpreferred work or activities.

- May not have *metacognition*, which is the awareness of one's thought process, and the ability to self-monitor and self-correct.

- May lack *self-direction* on the purpose and alignment of learning with postsecondary goals.

- May need *more leadership or guidance* on the purpose and value of the assessment(s) and how it benefits the BSSN.

- May need *accommodations*, such as extended time or audio presentation of the material.

BSSNs who may not value testing could benefit from added support strategies for motivation. Rewards for meeting expectations could be helpful, depending on the BSSN's unique profile. Be advised that some may not respond to the overuse of trick-for-treats found in some IEP methodologies. It is of critical importance to remember that assessments are for informational purposes only. They are a part of the BSSN's present level of performance, along with observable behaviors and informal classwork or measurements.

Homework

Homework is used to demonstrate understanding and is calculated in education expectations. However, BSSNs may need more emotional capacity or bandwidth, digital resources, or other supports at home to complete homework successfully as expected. Therefore, systems could change the weighting of grades. For example, instead of weighting 60% assessments, 30% homework, and 10% classwork/participation, a distribution of 50% classwork/participation, 30% assessments, and 20% homework may provide a more accurate assessment of the student's learning. Consider integrating alternative assessments, where students can demonstrate knowledge according to their preferred style or skill.

Transition Services

Transition services are an integral part of the education process and should be expected to begin toward the end of eighth grade. Parents should begin to explore skills, careers, or entrepreneurship opportunities when their child is around age nine. Several free and low-cost self-determination instruments are available to help young individuals make informed choices on their strengths and talents. BSSNs should begin to be included in transition discussions by age 14, or in eighth grade. If the BSSN is on an IEP, continuing the IEP should be discussed in the transition meeting from middle school to high school. By this time, BSSNs should be somewhat familiar with their IEP plans and can moderately participate in the transition meeting and plans. State vocational rehabilitation agencies (such as DORS in Maryland) help high school completers with disabilities to assess and prepare for employment access and success. Schools refer students to vocational rehabilitation agencies as part of the transition process.

Transition services also include goals to help BSSN connect language and social-emotional skills to the communication soft skills needed in the workplace.

Self-Directed

Self-directedness, or learner self-direction, refers to an individual's internal learning and growth process as well as the external influences experienced through instruction (Brockett & Hiemstra, 1991) Even though a BSSN might have a medical condition, gift, or disability, they may have been raised in a home where self-determination is a core value and may be motivated to succeed on their own terms. So, they may demonstrate a reluctance toward receiving services (even though they need them) or have a preference for how the service is delivered.

Female BSSNs, in particular, might also display confidence (and courteousness) in their communications about learning, which might present as cockiness in the classroom. "Self-directed learning is defined as the process of learning by which the individual establishes elements of control over their own learning and characteristics of learners, including self-efficacy and motivation" (Brockett, 1991), "Self-directed or self-regulated learning skills employ tenants of forethought, monitoring, control, and reaction in a learning transaction (Baumeister & Vohs, 2007) and encompass motivation or self-efficacy, strategic actions, and self-monitoring or correction, known as metacognition.

Getting BSSNs to Graduation or Completion

The national graduation rate for Black students is 80%, and for those with disabilities who graduated with a diploma, it is 72% and 11% for those with certificates (NCES, 2018-2019). Black students with disabilities are one and a half times more likely to drop out of school than white students with disabilities (NCES, 2017-2018). There are a few matters to consider that can help inspire academic completion for BSSN. In order to graduate, students must pass assessments and earn a prescribed type and amount of subject/course credits. Some states, like Maryland, also require volunteer service hours before graduation.

Decisions for choosing a certificate track vs. a diploma-track should be

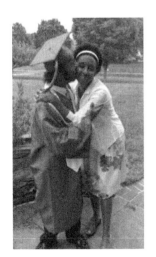

deferred until significant evidence of development is available and reviewed by parents and school team members. In most cases, deciding in early primary grades to place a child on an alternative assessment or certificate-bound track is too early. The BSSN should have the best possible chance to benefit from the academic opportunities present in the diploma-bound curriculum. As the IEP process is an annual review process with triennial evaluations, evaluation of the child's potential and placement is ongoing, and should always serve the child's best interests.

College and Workforce

People with disabilities are less likely to complete a bachelor's degree. There are college programs for students with disabilities. For example, in Maryland, Montgomery College has Developmental Education with a Graduate Transition Program led by longtime developmental education and inclusion champion Karla Nabors. McDaniel College in Maryland is intentional and proactive in servicing students with special learning needs.

Postsecondary experiences affect employment outcomes; a BSSN is also less likely to be employed. Below are disability unemployment rates:

- Blacks (21.6 %)
- Hispanics (16.1%)
- Whites (11.2 %)
- Asians (8.6 %)

(Bureau of Labor Statistics, 2015)

Utilized legal protections have helped to address disproportionality in a system normed in exclusivity. On June 29, 2023, after hearing *Students for Fair Admissions, Inc. v. President and Fellows of Harvard College*, the U.S. Supreme Court, voted six to three to overturn affirmative action in higher education admissions. The judgment to remove race as a preferred criterion for admission of qualified Blacks into higher education is expected to reduce Black student enrollment in Predominantly White Institutions (PWI) colleges and universities.

The absence of justice for educational inequity in higher education will affect BSSNs in secondary education. For example, the USC Race and Equity Center (University Southern California) posits that the racialized criterion removal will cause "interpretive overreach" across non-admissions departments which will universally defer to the ruling. So academic preparation programs or special education services, for example, would assume they, too, cannot affirm enrollment spaces specifically for Black students and deny race-specific services.

The 2023 SCOTUS decision on affirmative action in higher education could be a silver lining for some BSSN's. As one door closes, another may open the door to advance alternative pathways for skills in trades and entrepreneurship. A traditional life-skill path could yield more opportunities for Black students with special needs who have gifts, cognitive differences, social limitations, and developmental disabilities.

IDEA Disability Categories for RRIIPP Considerations

Disabilities are categorized to help make meaning for data collection, information, service provision, and other purposes. The exact definition of disabilities, as well as the different types or categories, may vary depending on the source and purpose of the information. For example, in the Developmental Driver Education program I designed in 2007 and led at Montgomery College, we defined our students as having social and cognitive limitations. Those whose impairment in giving and receiving signals in the context of driving is limited and, in that context, poses a threat to safety.

Below is a list of disabilities defined by IDEA for special education services. All students found eligible for special education services will be identified in the category with the most impact.

- Specific learning disability (SLD)
- Other health impairment (OHI)
- Autism spectrum disorder (ASD)
- Emotional disability (ED)
- Speech & language impairment (SLP)
- Visual impairment (VI)

- Deafness (DF)
- Hearing impairment (HI)
- Deaf-Blindness (DFB)
- Orthopedic impairment (OI)
- Intellectual disability (ID)
- Traumatic brain injury (TBI)
- Multiple disabilities (MD)

I firmly believe that had Korey Wise of the *Exonerated Central Park Five*, been appropriately RRIIPP'd from the pipeline of inequity; he may have been categorized under IDEA with hearing impairment a specific learning disability). Mr. Wise may not have been falsely accused or may not have been sentenced and served nine years in a penitentiary for a crime he did not commit.

Chapter Challenge: How might Korey Wise's life (or choose another adult) been different? Take a look back at the RRIIPP framework as you listen to his story, read the book, or see the movie: *When They See Us* by Ava DuVernay.

The identification of these disabilities for students in America, thankfully, comes with individualized services and supports to help students reach goals, use supplementary aids, and receive specialized therapies to improve their functioning in the school setting and for academic access. It is imperative that we clear the way for BSSNs to be appropriately identified and adequately serviced to experience success. May this text help you to provide better service for those BSSNs in your care.

Chapter 5

Synchronize Health and Education: Solutions for Referral, Diet, and Stigma

GOAL

Given evidence-based strategies of relationship-building, access to holistic care and nutrition, conscious bias redirection, and access to scientific research regarding natural remedies to treat and heal BSSN conditions and symptoms including dysfunctional and suicidal thoughts and impulsive behaviors, and applied with fidelity, stakeholders will synchronize health and education for BSSNs, by (e.g. March 2026) as measured by records of results in five out of seven reviews.

Introduction: This chapter offers insights into how health intersects with education for Black students with special needs. Health practitioners including doctors, therapists, psychiatrists, surgeons, and psychologists, play a key role in the diagnosis, referral, and treatment of the medical conditions of BSSNs. Teachers, administrators, counselors, and related service providers can administer education plans in school settings with consideration of recommendations from health practitioners. BSSN parents are often stuck in the middle, challenged on the one end by health disparity, and education disparity on the other end. Instead of siloed sectors, this chapter calls for synchronicity in evaluation, treatment, and well-being.

Policy Positions

After the unrest and demand for racial justice exploded in 2020, and recognizing the need to declare a stance on equity and unity with marginalized people, several organizations have modified or created position statements. The American Academy of Pediatrics offers us an example. In 2019, the AAP released a policy statement entitled, *The Impact of Racism on Child and Adolescent Health*. The statement leveraged the declaration of social determination by the World Health Organization to showcase the victimization of racialized groups by racism in healthcare, mental, and maternal health in particular. The following is an excerpt from the AAP public policy statement. As you read this chapter, keep this description of the relationship between racism and health in mind. After the chapter, you will be asked to reflect.

> *Racism is a core social determinant of health that drives health inequities. The World Health Organization defines social determinants of health as "the conditions in which people are born, grow, live, work, and age." These determinants are influenced by economic, political, and social factors linked to health inequities (avoidable inequalities in health between groups of people within populations and between countries). These health inequities are not the result of individual behavior choices or genetic predisposition but are caused by economic, political, and social conditions, including racism.*
>
> *The impact of racism has been linked to birth disparities and mental health problems in children and adolescents. The biological mechanism that emerges from chronic stress leads to increased and prolonged exposure to stress hormones and oxidative stress at the cellular level. Prolonged exposure to stress hormones, such as cortisol, leads to inflammatory reactions predisposing individuals to chronic disease. For example, racial disparities in the infant mortality rate remain, and the complications of low birth weight have been associated with perceived racial discrimination and maternal stress. (Trent et al., 2019)*

You Hold the Keys

In a study of nine- to twelve-year-olds, thirty-eight children were compared to adults to recognize how the brain works as it develops mature inhibitory control. Inhibitory control is the "...ability to adaptively and flexibly control one's actions, including inhibiting prepotent, but inappropriate, responses in favor of goal-directed behavior, (which) is critical for cognitive and affective development" (source needed). In short, the ability to start/go and end/stop is critical for human development and functioning. In his Parent-Child Journey parent education workshops and books, Dr. Dan Shapiro illustrates this start-stop conundrum. Poor inhibitory action control in childhood is a hallmark of neurodevelopmental disorders, including attention-deficit/hyperactivity disorder (ADHD) and autism spectrum disorder (Cai et al., 2019).

Conversely, children with better inhibitory control abilities tend to have better academic performance and emotion regulation skills. BSSNs with inhibitory control are less likely to engage in maladaptive behaviors that are self-destructive. Children without adult-like brain maturity responses, such as those with developmental disorders and disabilities, will struggle with inhibitory control and be less able to use the start-stop key/function, in comparison to their neurotypical peers.

Increase Nutrition

We know adequate school nutrition is linked to improved literacy and math scores, improved cognitive function, reduced absenteeism, and long-term positive educational outcomes. Nutrition as a part of a holistic treatment plan and practical application can be considered through the family physician and family-school partnership. Ensuring adequate nutrition for BSSNs with disabilities often requires more planning for special diets. According to a study on the oligoantigenic diet (one that avoids certain foods that often trigger allergies or intolerances), "Personalized nutrition could be a useful tool for the personalized treatment of ADHD symptoms" (Walz, et al., 2022)

Given that "subthreshold (vs. full syndrome disorders) juvenile ADHD is a risk factor for addiction disorders and impaired social interactions in adults" (Shankman et al., 2009), food addiction is a warning to heed.

> *While "chocolate may balance low levels of mood regulation including serotonin and dopamine," according to the Journal of the American Dietetic Association (year?), refined sugar is not so beneficial. The World Health Organization (WHO) recommends less than 10% of added or free sugars per daily caloric intake, to avoid "negative effects of excessive or prolonged sugar intake." (Gillespie et al., 2023)*

> *There is also the potential for sugar-associated impairments, particularly regarding impacts on cognition and developmental conditions, that impose a greater challenge for those with an underlying predisposition (e.g., a mental health condition) or an existing condition (such as ADHD). (Gillespie et al., 2023)*

Early research on rats from Princeton University found that sugar is more addictive than substances such as cocaine, causing withdrawal symptoms such as depression and behavioral problems when addicts try cutting out sugar completely (NIH 2002, 2008). More on sugar later in this chapter.

Water Is Chief

Water is necessary for all life, "The chief thing for life is water" (Sirach 29:21). The human body is upwards of three-quarters water, (approximately 60%) and serves as a solvent, acts as a building material, and carries nutrients and waste products (Jéquier, 2010). As emphasized in the European Journal of Clinical Nutrition, "the regulation of water balance is essential for the maintenance of health and life." (Jéquier, 2010). Contrary to the common promotion of alternatives, "water is

the only liquid nutrient that is really essential for body hydration" (Jéquier, 2010). Using the measure of an eight-ounce cup, drinking standards from the CDC for children are as follows:
- 5-8 years of age: 5 cups daily (or > 40 oz per day),
- 9-12 years of age: 7 cups daily (or > 56 oz per day).
- 13 and older: 8-10 cups daily (or > 64oz)

Certain factors, such as medical conditions and sex will cause variation in the recommendations.

Water impacts learning and health for BSSNs. Water is an essential nutrient that has "a role in overall bodily system functioning (e.g., cognition) and in the prevention of chronic conditions and diseases common in the 21st century such as obesity and tooth decay." (Pivarnik, et al. 1994). I asked a school nurse with over 20 years of experience about water for BSSNs in school and she said that the children "are not drinking enough water" and that "water plays a huge role in diabetes management because it helps to dilute blood glucose." According to the National Library of Medicine, "Children and adolescents are not consuming enough water, instead opting for sugar-sweetened beverages (sodas, sports and energy drinks, milks, coffees, and fruit-flavored drinks with added sugars), 100% fruit juice, and other beverages." Drinking sufficient amounts of water can lead to improved weight status, reduced dental caries, and improved cognition among children and adolescents" (Patal, et al., 2011)

According to CDC.org, about half of all school-aged children are underhydrated. The American Journal of Public Health, cites that, "The prevalence of inadequate hydration or underhydration was 54.5%, and that the odds of inadequate hydration were 1.76 times higher among boys than girls and 1.34 times higher among non-Hispanic Blacks than non-Hispanic Whites" (Kenney, et al. 2015). According to a 2018 literature review and meta-analysis on dehydration's relationship with cognitive performance, it was found that "Despite variability among studies, dehydration impairs cognitive performance, particularly for tasks involving attention, executive function, and motor coordination when water deficits exceed 2% body mass loss" (Wittbrodt, et al. 2018). The study observed that "...tasks requiring attention and/or executive function were significantly more impaired after dehydration, while others (e.g., information processing, memory, reaction time tasks) were not" (Wittbrodt, et al. 2018).

Water Intake Recommendations

Water can be a difference maker for many BSSNs. However, there are a few considerations to make before you 'pour the water':

- **Make sure the water has minerals.** Natural Mineral Water has salts that are beneficial for the body's pH balance (Quattrini, et al., 2016), and having the right balance helps maintain and regulate the amount of water in the cells. The "salt in our bodies is also important because it contains electrolytes—minerals such as sodium, potassium, and chloride—that carry an electrical charge through the blood and body fluids, keeping hydration at a healthy level."(nationalgeographic.com) Without the electrolytes by way of salt, hyponatremia sets in causing dizziness, confusion, flu-like sickness, and sleep problems as some examples.

- **Medications and medical conditions.** Know which medications might interfere with the body's natural ability to hydrate. Medications that make the heat more dangerous include certain anti-depressants, diuretics, and blood pressure medicine, which can interfere with kidney function and electrolyte levels. People with diabetes, which already increases the need to urinate, need to closely monitor fluid intake *(nationalgeographic.com)*.

- **Measure the right amount of water.** Target above the minimum recommendation but not too much. Providing servings of between 300 and 500 milliliters (about 10-16.8 fl.oz) of water to children during the school day has been shown to improve cognitive performance and mood. (Kenney, et al., 2015). At the other end of the spectrum is water intoxication which can lead to hyponatremia also known as low blood sodium and occurs when too much water is consumed too rapidly. Drinking excessive amounts of water can overwhelm your kidneys and dilute the sodium content of your blood. Symptoms include headaches, fatigue, and nausea. (Mayo Clinic, 2022).

- **Market positively water intake and water education resources.** Schools can help kids stay hydrated by promoting water access, changing school wellness policies, and involving community partners, students, and parents (CDC, 2022). CDC Healthy Schools has developed modules that discuss resources to help schools: Ensure water is safe, promote water as an ideal beverage choice, make clean and free drinking water easily available in different areas of the school, and meet the free drinking water requirements in the National School Lunch Program and the School Breakfast Program, at minimum (CDC, 2022).

- **Monitor water safety.** Check that the water is free of lead and other contaminants. Lead can cause brain damage to children at levels too low to cause clinically evident signs and symptoms. Research has linked lead toxicity levels to learning disabilities, poor classroom performance, and increased aggression. Lead exposure also causes anemia, hypertension, renal impairment, immunotoxicity, and toxicity to the reproductive organs (EducationWeek, 2019).

"Although schools participating in the National School Lunch Program must provide free drinking water during meals, implementation varies, and many school districts struggles with older infrastructure that limit their capacity to provide safe drinking water." (CDC). Access to clean water is not universal. While 92 percent of the population supplied by community water systems receives drinking water that meets all health-based standards all of the time, according to the Clean Water Act (CWA), which establishes the basic structure for regulating discharges of pollutants into the waters of the United States and regulating quality standards for surface waters, there are an estimated nine million lead service lines in need of replacement across the US (EPA, 2024) According to the EPA website, grants are earmarked for Voluntary Lead Testing in Schools and Child Care and for Assistance for Small and Disadvantaged Communities for lead testing and compliance improvements according to the SDWA. Schools across the country have found elevated lead levels in drinking water.

In 2014 alarmingly high levels of lead were found in the Flint Michigan water system and in lead-based paint. In Flint, "...families drank, bathed, and cooked in their homes with lead-laced water from the Flint River for 17 months before the problem was discovered and the water supply was shut off" (EdWeek, 2019). According to WHO (World Health Organization), lead can affect children's brain development, resulting in reduced intelligence quotient (IQ), behavioral changes such as reduced attention span and increased antisocial behavior, and reduced educational attainment. The superintendent reported that the "percentage of special education students has increased by 56 percent, rising from 13.1% in 2012-13—the school year before the water crisis began—to 20.5%" in 2018. "…28% of the district's students have individualized education programs…more than double the national average…" (EdWeek, 2019). Ten years later, the Drinking Water Division of the Michigan Department of Environment, Great Lakes and Energy reported to

NPR news that, "tests of Flint's tap water continue to show the presence of lead, but the levels are within federal and state standards" (Carmody, 2024).

Water Source Examples

Water in the Air

Atmospheric Water Generators (AWGs), extract water vapor from the air similarly to how a dehumidifier works. Retired U.S. Army officer Moses West invented a community sized AWG that he dubbed the "green machine" that collects water out of the air for drinking and other uses. His AWG is capable of providing clean water just about anywhere in the world and is already globally being used by the armed forces of the United States, has served four water-stressed countries, and many urban and rural areas in America (moseswestfoundation.org, 2023). In 2019, Mr. West placed an ASW unit in Flint, Michigan to combat the horrific lead-contamination tragedy where it provided between 1,200 and 2,000 gallons of water daily. However, after only a week, the unit was sabotaged, rendering it temporarily inoperable. During an interview with WNEM TV5 in 2019, Moses speculated that the kind of damage done to the unit was too detailed and intricate to be the work of a novice. He mused out loud that "Giving thousands of gallons of water away free is costing someone a lot of money." (McCrary, 2019)

The Moses West Foundation has given six million gallons and counting of clean water to people around the world.

Water Out of the Rock

One spring day, on a family outing a two-and-a-half-hour drive to a national park culminating with a drive up a mountain, we saw several cars pulled over on the opposite side of the road. There were a few people with large containers waiting patiently, and surprisingly, we saw water flowing down the mountainside through two narrow PVC pipes. It was easily accessible so drivers could drink to their heart's content or fill up their water containers (hopefully not plastic) with FREE fresh, cool, mineral-rich H2O. We stopped for a drink, and it was the best water I had tasted since my taste buds were satiated by a steady flow of water near the Banias Waterfall in Israel. (In some countries people walk for dirty water the same distance we had just driven and they are thankful for it.) A year later we returned to that same place excited to share our discovery with other family members. Unbeknownst to me, just on the other side of the road down behind the guardrail was a PVC pipe with a circumference ten times the size of the aforementioned pipe. It had so many gallons pouring out we could have not only drank but actually showered under it. How interesting that we were satisfied with the amount of the resource given, when all the while, the water flowed in abundance behind a barrier. We were happy and satisfied as if we had found a gold nugget, when in reality a few feet away there was actually a goldmine, a waterfall pouring out water to those who had access to the great resource because they were on the other side of the barrier.

War on Drugs

In 2016, Former President Richard Nixon's Domestic Policy Advisor, John Erlichman, revealed in *Harper's Magazine* that the War on Drugs that began in the 1960s was initiated in part as a racially motivated "crusade" to criminalize blacks (Baum, 2016). The audiotape of this admission was finally released from the National Archives of an October 1971 conversation between President Nixon and the then-Governor of California and future president, Ronald Reagan, after being withheld in 2000 to protect Reagan's privacy. According to a July 2019 article in *The Atlantic* by Tim Naftali, the first director of the Richard Nixon Presidential Library and Museum, as he reported, the audio revealed Reagan had referred to UN African delegates as "monkeys" saying, "damn them, they're still uncomfortable wearing shoes!" as President Nixon laughingly responded saying "the tail was wagging the dog" (Naftali, 2019). Nixon candidly disclosed his views on Africans and African

Americans to his former aid, Harvard professor Daniel Patrick Moynihan, divulging his attraction to theories linking IQ to race and looking for Moynihan's views. Nixon believed in a hierarchy of races, believing Whites and Asians to be vastly superior to Blacks and Latinos. This and other behaviors betray that Nixon allowed his racism to shape U.S. policies, including welfare, school busing, and the horrific war on drugs (The Atlantic, 2019)

Fast forwarding to the 1980s, President Ronald Reagan waged his own version of the War on Drugs (crack), which in hindsight now appears to be a cleverly veiled continuation of President Nixon's insidiously concealed war on Blacks. Reagan's war yielded much fruit in the form of unprecedented violence, murder, and the accelerated massive incarceration of Blacks fueled by new congressional bills, such as The Comprehensive Crime Control Act and the Anti-Drug Abuse Act, summarized below.

The Comprehensive Crime Control Act was introduced in the U.S. House of Representatives on February 9, 1984. The bill's tenets covered bail, sentencing reform, the insanity defense, penalties for drug law offenses, prosecution of certain minors as adults, and many other statutes (www.OJP.gov, 2022), adversely overhauling the federal parole system.

Anti-Drug Abuse Act of 1986. The bill consisted of 15 titles beginning with Anti-Drug enforcement, covering narcotics penalties, assets forfeiture, labeling of controlled substances and more. (U.S. Department of Justice, Office of Justice Programs 1986) This introduced the notorious 100-to-1 ratio relating to the amount of crack versus powder cocaine needed to trigger mandatory minimum prison sentences, meaning that Blacks in possession of *five grams of crack cocaine* mandated the same minimum sentence as White offenders in possession of *500 grams of powder cocaine.* (ACLU, 2007)

The effects of the more than twenty-year campaign may still be impacting an untold number of Blacks (including BSSNs) with an incarcerated family member(s) who served long sentences. As of 2018, 80.0% of crack cocaine trafficking offenders were Black (CDC, 2018). These policies distributed an unbalanced allocation of funding to law enforcement while withholding monies from prevention, intervention, and treatment.

Opioid Crisis

Comparatively, the opioid crisis of the 2020s, "was initially approached as a rural problem impacting a White/Caucasian demographic" (Gondré-Lewis et al., 2022) and rolled out the red carpet with September 21 as National Opioid and Substance Awareness Day and a compassionate rapid response of treatment and recovery, while inundating communities and schools with sympathetic campaigns. Campaigns like the National Opioid Action Coalition's (NOAC) Power of One, proclaim that "Each of us has a role in the fight against opioid MISUSE"—a notable difference from the language of ABUSE, in the War on Drugs.

Power of One encouraged each individual to: (a) Participate in a take-back program and get rid of the unneeded opioids in the home; (b) Help set up a voluntary community education program; (c) Coach kids on the risks of opioids; (d)Sponsor someone in recovery looking for a job; or to ask a government leader for more treatment resources (nationalopioidactioncoalition.org).

War on Sugar

Comprehensive strategies designed for a targeted audience with a targeted substance is possible. What if, for the benefit of BSSNs health, the crisis stratagems in the allocation of financial and human resources of the former War on Drugs along with the information and medical resources of the rapid response opioid methodology, were used to mitigate the devastating effects of the overuse of refined added sugar?

According to the CDC's Dietary Guidelines for Americans, people older than two years should keep sugars to less than 10% of their total daily calories. This, however, can be a daunting task, as added sugars are often hidden in an array of other names, like fructose, dextrose, cane juice, fruit nectars, glucose, high-fructose, corn syrup, honey, lactose, malt syrup, maltose, molasses, and sucrose (cdc.gov). This is very concerning if we consider how much for BSSNs these sweeteners dominate the percentage of calories at breakfast, lunch, dinner, and snacks in amounts that far exceed these healthy recommendations. "There is enough evidence to say elevated sugar consumption is an important contributor to weight gain" (Johns Hopkins, 2023).

Childhood obesity among black children ages 2–19 years old was 24.8% leading to obesity-related conditions including high blood pressure, high cholesterol, Type 2 diabetes, breathing problems such as asthma and sleep apnea, and joint problems. (CDC National Center for Health Statistics 2017-2020 cdc.gov)

Children in utero can be affected by the things we ingest and digest. For example, alcohol is widely known to affect the unborn child's brain, causing developmental disabilities collectively termed FASD: Fetal Alcohol Spectrum Disorders. When alcohol is consumed, it dehydrates the largest organ in the body, the skin, depriving it of vitamins and nutrients. Overconsumption of ethanol/alcohol plays a leading role in obesity, related maladies like Type 2 diabetes, and fatty liver disease (Lustig, 2010). Nowadays, children are getting alcohol-related diseases without the consumption of alcohol (Lustig, 2010). Might sugar be the new alcohol? A 2010 study in the Journal of the American Dietetic Association revealed that it can lead to a "vicious cycle of excessive consumption and disease consistent with metabolic syndrome. (Lustig, 2010). We would not want our BSSNs to abuse alcohol due to the health risks and dangers, yet we are seeing the same conditions in those who overindulge in sugar.

The market Considering this contributory relationship between over-consumption of added sugars and disease, it should be illegal for corporate structures to distribute to community systems an endless supply of refined sugar cane and its substitutes to Black children under the age of 18. Where is the "War on Sugar"? Where are the Public Service Announcements (PSAs) and the information fairs at schools on the mind-altering effects of excess refined cane sugar and its connection to these health risks? Why is added refined sugar so readily available in school for breakfast and lunches? What are the adult models eating in the presence of the Black children? The American Heart Association recommends limiting added sugar to nine teaspoons (36 grams) daily for most men and six teaspoons (25 grams) daily for women; the average adult gets about 17 teaspoons daily, almost doubling the limit for men and tripling the limit for women (Merschel, 2023).

A sugar study on adults published in 2023 by the American Journal of Clinical Nutrition found that fructose from added sugar and juice was positively associated with the risk of coronary heart disease; fructose from fruits and vegetables was not. (Dennis, et al., 2023) If BSSNs are hydrating with fruit and sports drinks, "switching to water might help…avoid 35 grams of added sugar (nearly 9 teaspoons) per 20-ounce bottle." (Merschel, 2023). Water as a remedy, what a novel idea; it is essential for bodily systems to function properly.

If we were to adopt the same opioid stratagem, free rescue remedies would be administered by school nurses and pharmacies would offer detoxification and unrefined sugar replacements. Can you envision the campaign toward transformation? Taking hold of nutrition in home-packed and school provided breakfasts and lunches is critical for academic success. The Education Trust advocates that "adequate school nutrition is linked to improved literacy and math scores, improved cognitive function, reduced absenteeism, and long-term positive educational outcomes" in its 2022 Child Nutrition Reauthorization-Recommendations for Congress (EdTrust.org, 2022).

There are assumptions that parents carry the blame for some disabilities, such as ADHD or ASD. Our attention is better served by turning toward a healthy lifestyle, instead of parents self-flagellating or beating themselves up about the role they may have played in contributing to a disability (if at all possible) in utero. Genetics show us our potential for disease, but diet, nutrition, environment, and lifestyle awaken disease and health that might otherwise remain dormant. Nutrition guidance from federal studies, medical experts, and naturopaths all recommend diets rich in green leafy vegetables, healthy fats found in nuts and avocados, oils such as olive and coconut, and fish. Fish with fins and scales, such as wild-caught salmon and light tuna, contain lower levels of mercury, a deadly neurotoxin. The scales on the fish provide a barrier, almost like an armor, against pathogens.

Reduce Food Insecurity

Health and education are interdependent and highly variable in the practices and policies that affect BSSNs. The relationship between nutrition and learning is clearly linked, and food insecurity is the corrosion damaging BSSN potential. The USDA defines food insecurity as the lack of consistent access to enough food, even temporarily, for every person in a household to live an active, healthy life.

According to The Education Trust,

> *. . . too many students—especially Black students, Latino students, and students from low-income backgrounds—are still experiencing food insecurity in our nation. People of color are more likely to live in food deserts, and, as a result, many students do not have access to the necessary nutrition for their physical, mental, socioemotional, and academic growth. During the COVID-19 pandemic, food insecurity among Black and Latino households with children skyrocketed, leaving nearly 4 in 10 families struggling to feed their families.*

- *8% of African Americans live in a census tract with a supermarket, compared to 31% of Whites.*
- *Low-income zip codes have 30% more convenience stores, which tend to lack healthy items, than middle-income ZIP codes.*

According to Learning For Justice, 2022:

> *These convenience stores and fast-food restaurants do not typically sell the variety of foods needed for a healthy diet such as fresh fruits and vegetables, whole grains, fresh dairy, and lean meat products. If they do sell them, they often cost more than they cost at grocery stores. The limited options put those who live in food deserts at a financial and nutritional disadvantage.*

BSSNs are at a nutritional disadvantage because of food insecurity. According to Feeding America, living with a disability or chronic condition may lead to higher medical costs, prevent people (like parents of BSSNs) from working regularly, or make quality food unaffordable. Food insecurity is also an economic issue, and Black families are at 15% of the median and mean wealth of White families according to the Federal Reserve System in 2019. The typical White family has eight times the wealth of the typical Black family and five times the wealth of the typical Hispanic (Latinx) family (Board of Governors of the Federal Reserve System, 2019) In dollars and cents, that is a reported median comparison of $24K to $188K, and a mean of $142K to $983K for Black to White wealth.

The decision for parents of BSSNs to consistently make critical choices of housing or medicine over food is a clear and present reality. While charity meet needs, they are not sustainable. For food desert areas, practices such as creating community farming systems (e.g. Urban Gardens in Milwaukee, Wisconsin), and investing in community development properties (e.g. Impact Change in Rock Hill, South Carolina) are more effective and are beginning to make a difference.

Increase Natural Remedies

Many BSSN mothers move as lionesses, on the hunt for the root causes of developmental behaviors and their triggers, and remedies ranging from what grandma and auntie used to the latest in neuroscientific research. When used correctly, natural remedies, including herbs or apothecary applications, work with or service the body to heal conditions without damaging the other systems' functioning properties. For example, whole plants possess abundant active components, creating balance and equilibrium; the body generally knows how to respond to whole-plant medicine. While natural remedies are intuitive, medications are necessary in certain cases.

Conventional/pharmacological applications, by design, mitigate the symptoms of the condition, accompanied by a host of reported side-effects to other body parts varying in degrees from mild to severe. Costs of medications, with and without insurance, can exceed even the most well-thought-out BSSN family budget. Natural remedies, simplified diet, exercise, or readily available herbs can be much easier on the wallet.

More BSSN parents are interested in using natural remedies, such as herbology or homeopathy, and seek standardized protocols or administration providers. Dr. Shapiro says, "There should not be a divide between pharmacology and natural remedies; both should be subjected to the same scientific analysis." He says they should all be applied with the scientific method, with the source of the product determining its safety or effectiveness. He says some natural and unnatural materials are "wonderful, effective, and safe."

Several studies have been administered on the effectiveness of biochemical dietary eliminations. Identifying food intolerances and allergic reactions and eliminating food-based toxins and environmental chemicals are strategies associated with the Oligoantigenic diet.

One example of an herbal remedy vigorously studied on children under 12 years has been the valerian root/lemon balm combination for treating ADHD symptoms. Clinical trial reports that the combination reduced symptoms of restlessness and insomnia, improving concentration and alleviating insomnia and restlessness. A European study on valerian and lemon balm reported that,

> *The fraction of children having strong symptoms of poor ability to focus decreased from 75% to 14%, hyperactivity from 61% to 13%, and impulsiveness from 59% to 22%. In addition, parent-rated social behavior, sleep, and symptom burden showed highly significant improvements (Gromball, et al., 2014).*

Studies such as this reveal the opportunities to explore accessible alternatives for parents of BSSNs as they desperately seek solutions.

Stigma, Bias, Trauma & Medicine: Barriers to Accessing Care

Dr. Shapiro says that. particularly in the greater Washington, DC area, access to psychiatric care and stigma is "a challenge in many communities" and "both are huge problems." For Shapiro, minorities are not unique in how they receive care; it is more about access to it. He says that before he retired from practice, he offered a sliding scale fee, and there had been more diversity, so he was "really pleased." The percentage of his Black or Latinx practice was in the 10-20% range. He says that Spanish-speaking families tend to be college graduates with a higher socioeconomic status than Black families.

Reduce Stigma

Stigma is "a set of negative and unfair beliefs that a society or group of people have about something" (Merriam-Webster Dictionary). I would say this more strongly: Stigma is prejudice or negative stereotyping that often results in discriminatory action. The stigma of being disabled was, by the Surgeon General in 1999, considered "the most formidable obstacle to future progress in the arena of mental illness and health" (U.S. Department of Health and Human Services, 1999, p. 3). Many BSSNs, are doubly stigmatized with the co-occurrence of belonging to a racially marginalized group membership and having a psychiatric illness. Double stigmas may lead to delayed or aborted treatment, increased mortality and morbidity, decreased well-being, and increased psychiatric symptomatology. (Gary, 2005). Socioeconomic status is a determinant of stigma. Higher levels of education signify the ability to achieve goals and realize hopes. The more hopes and dreams, for example, college-bound or entrepreneur bound, the more compelled BSSNs are to address developmental barriers to maintain their place in a higher socioeconomic class.

Dr. Shapiro says that while "Stigma is there for mental health and developmental disabilities," He also sees significant differences in how Black and Latinx families view disability and approach treatment. "Black families are interested in pursuing care–they see it, but there is no trust, whereas Latinx families are harder to get in the door." He has worked to make his free virtual group training programs for parents accessible. For example, he said that he worked with a community and language consultant from Spain to provide information from English to Spanish. He said, "We've translated materials into Spanish and hit the Spanish (speaking) community hard, (yet)—-zero registrations, whereas the Black families will come in good numbers."

One of the many things I learned from being director of the Hispanic Business and Training Institute at our community college is the value of authenticity for the Latinx community. Authenticity is held in high regard within ethnic communities. It is not enough to translate something into Spanish (and if you do, you had better make sure it is the proper dialect because European Spanish is not the same as Latin American Spanish) or speak to someone in Spanish. Trust is always on trial when in relationship with communities not your own. It did not matter that my grandfather was "part" Mexican, or that I had "friends who were Latinx," or that I was well-meaning, or that we had Spanish-speaking team members. While I know that the Latinx community benefited from the learning programs and services we provided, I did not get the engagement and connection I hoped for because of my language limitation.

Reduce Physician Racial Bias

Parents call them children. Doctors call them patients. Teachers call them students. These professionals all provide care for our BSSNs. To best help our BSSNs it is important to develop stronger relationships between parents, physicians or therapists, and teachers. Dr. Joette James and I developed and shared a powerful presentation to physicians on the topic of bias and referral that outlined the role of the physicians in the process of referrals and assessment for BSSNs (see RRIIPP Chapter Four for reference).

Research indicates that discrimination through IQ testing, specifically, has contributed to the disproportional placement of African American children in special education (Affeldt, 2000). The 1979 *Larry P vs. Riles* case precedent in California specifically prohibited using standardized IQ tests solely to diagnose Intellectual Disability. Appropriately applying the I (Identification) in the **RRIIPP** framework clarifies the need to use multiple data sources in disability determinations. Black/African American children are underrepresented in standardization samples, and research on test bias is lacking (i.e., psychometric properties of tests) (James & Jackson, 2021).

Recognizing stereotypes and related mindsets are relevant in the work to correct the disparities in health and education. Particularly, understanding stereotype threat can help us work through stigma, and address over- and underidentification. Stereotype threat is defined as, "being at risk of confirming, as self-characteristic, a negative stereotype about one's group" (Steele et. al., 1995). Once, a school team proposed to not evaluate a BSSN for impact of hyperactivity on learning because, "Black boys are overidentified for ADHD," as defended by the Black school psychologist.

Stereotype Threat:

- Defined as the fear of being judged based on a negative stereotype of a person's specific group.
- Multiple studies have documented this phenomenon in IQ, neuropsychological testing, math, and work performance.
- The strength of racial identity may be a moderator of the effect.
- Research has shown higher levels of test-taking anxiety in African American middle school students and more test-taking behaviors indicating anxiety (e.g., more answer-changing during test-taking).

The language used in evaluation reporting should be unbiased and culturally competent. Parents should review reports before dis-seminating them to various professionals and schools. Parents can ask for edits and redactions as applicable.

Question for Thought:

How might disproportionality in under-identification and Stereotype Threat be related?

Reduce Trauma

In order to overcome trauma, we must increase trust within families and communities. The work of Pace Community Facilitators helps to share resources and information related to trauma. They share stories, research, and resources related to trauma for families. Most importantly, they help to keep families and leaders aware of the ten Adverse Childhood Experiences or ACES that affect long-term (and acute) health. Given the expansive trauma from oppression, systemic racism, and limited agency across the Black community, the likelihood of having multiple ACES for BSSNs is high.

See the list of the ten (10) Adverse Childhood Experiences (ACEs):

- Physical abuse
- Sexual abuse
- Verbal abuse
- Physical neglect
- Emotional neglect
- A family member who is depressed or diagnosed with other mental illness
- A family member who is addicted to alcohol or another substance
- A family member who is in prison
- Witnessing a mother being abused
- Losing a parent to separation, divorce, or death.

Medical and disability professionals, when making a disability diagnosis, should evaluate for ACES and trauma. The more adverse experiences the BSSN has, the greater potential for disease and poor health which impact learning. Through education— a free and appropriate education

---

How many of the ten (10) ACES (Adverse Childhood Experiences) were a part of your childhood?

How many of the ten (10) ACEs has your BSSN experienced?

with fidelity and meaningful progress— there is an opportunity to overcome the trauma from one's past.

NAMI, the National Alliance on Mental Illness, found that "racial and ethnic minorities receive lower-quality health care than white people— even when insurance status, income, age, and severity of conditions are comparable" (Reference). Since the 2003 recommendation for culturally relevant research studies (Smedley et al., 2003), there continue to be improvements in exploring addressing health inequities, stigma, and trauma. For example, pediatrician Joe Wright wrote the 2022 AAP Policy Statement, Eliminating Race-Based Medicine, to remove the socially constructed race factor from pediatric medicine (Wright, et al., 2022).

Consider the Biopsychosocial Model of Health

Just as there is no one cause of a developmental disability, there is no one solution for improving life quality. Families not well-steeped in knowledge about the biology of developmental differences will be disadvantaged. "Prepare the child for the road and prepare the road for the child," says Dr. Dan Shapiro. Biology, sociology, and psychology domains must be routinely and adequately attended to across all environments. Biology refers to the medical factors of the disability, Sociology addresses the social and cultural aspects of the disability, and Psychological pertains to the emotional and educational performances of the disability.

We find these three domains in the joint policy statement of The Arc and the AAIDD (American Association on Intellectual and Developmental Disabilities), "Valuing the lives, diversity, and contributions of people with IDD (Intellectual Disabilities) and advancing policies that mitigate the impact of psychoeducational, sociocultural, biomedical, and justice causes of disability are compatible positions." BSSNs who have IDD or DD would best be prepared by home and school environments that optimize biopsychosocial practices and policies.

Dr. Dan Shapiro says that the degree or perception of impairment largely depends upon/within the culture you live in. So, if your society's social context is based upon some over-affirmation of advanced functioning, inordinate parental pressure, or hyperintelligence, then the recognition of those with impairments will be glaring, and those with developmental disabilities will feel isolated. If, however, your society's context values creativity, diversity, compassion, and community, then BSSNs with developmental disabilities will be appreciated and included.

Let us take Sarah, for example, a student with dyslexia: a language-based developmental disability. At home, where she lives with her loving father, mother, and siblings, she is called "brilliant." In school, with far more typically developing peers, she's considered "learning disabled." In her music class, where her talents are valued, she's called "neurodiverse." So, which is it?

Healthy environments such as home and school can facilitate healthy activities and coping skills. For students with developmental differences and disabilities, teams should adopt goals for coping skills by the school psychologist using any supplementary aids and services that are known to be effective. Responsible parenting can nurture belonging at home with family and friends through regular family meals and meetings. These meaningful interactions help reinforce resilience when BSSNs encounter situations outside of home. Responsible parenting also involves treating illness and engaging the appropriate, unbiased healthcare professional or physician.

Treatment of illness can be an aspect of a holistic treatment plan. It is important to note that while psychological therapy is part of a holistic treatment plan (and an evidence-based intervention), "Healing is therapeutic; but not all therapy is healing," as California State University President, Dr. Thomas Parham, proclaimed. Dr. Parham describes his approach to working with African American clients as integrating spirituality, interconnectedness, and self-knowledge. Spirituality as part of therapy varies. According to Pew Research Center, nearly half of Black Americans "believe that God or a higher power talks to them directly" (Faith Among Black Americans, 2021).

It is no secret the enslaved, in serving their oppressors in a strange land, were forced to abandon much of their heritage and traditions. The faith of those enslaved and oppressed is what fueled their resilience, and it still holds that power today for many of their descendants. It resonates in artifacts like *Slave Songs of the United States*, a compilation of 136 negro spiritual songs with music and lyrics including *Roll Jordan Roll, Michael Row Your Boat Ashore,* and *I Heard from Heaven Today, which* expressed a hope of being redeemed in eternal life (Allen et. al., 1867). The transgenerational hope continues. Emerging is the decolonization of the traditional mental health treatment. Practitioners are changing how mental health is treated, bringing forward affirmation of culture and faith.

Parents are encouraged to not deny psychological services, but rather help shape the form of those services. One way is to differentiate psychological services in the school from private therapy. In school, psychological services are generally purposed to support the IEP social-emotional goals in the form of counseling sessions, for example. Whereas in private therapy, the therapy is broader and can usually target topics by parent choice and child need which extend beyond school. Choosing a private therapist with cultural competence, respect for parental authority, regard for spiritual practices, and relatability to the child is a valuable task for the BSSN parent. It is also the choice of the BSSN parent to share the progress notes of the private therapy provider with the school-based psychologist.

> Reflection Questions (Choose one or both)
>
> In your practice, what are some ways you provide BSSN parents with voice or agency in your delivery of services with the BSSN?
>
> Reread the excerpt from the 2019 American Academy of Pediatrics policy statement above entitled, *The Impact of Racism on Child and Adolescent Health*. Identify and explain how a practice or policy insight from this chapter for BSSNs is most relevant to the excerpt?

Chapter 6

Educational Leadership for Parents and Professionals

GOALS

Given *RRIIPP* and *Educational Leadership for Parents*© training, practices, and modeling, parents of BSSNs will be able to recognize their child's difference, disability, or gift, develop a plan to collaboratively advocate for their child, and monitor the plans for meaningful progress for at least one BSSN by (e.g. June 2026), as measured by appropriate identification, placement, at least two areas of progress.

Given *RRIIPP* and *Identifying and Removing Obstacles for Black Students with Special Needs*© training, educators will be able to appropriately refer and apply a proper response to intervention (RTI) for at least two BSSNs by (e.g. March 2026) as measured by student progress in reading or math, and parent satisfaction record.

Given RTI (Response To Intervention), evidence-based training and case conferences, special education teams will be able to appropriately identify, mitigate disciplinary action, and validate appropriate placement for at least five BSSNs by (e.g. June 2026), as measured by BSSN progress and leveled advancement in social-emotional, academic, and adaptive impact areas, and parent satisfaction record.

CHAPTER INTRODUCTION

This chapter defines educational leadership and provides professional development for educators and service providers in both general and special education. Professional development such as cultural competence, advocacy, and collaboration is emphasized. The chapter also boldly recommends the extension of the discipline of educational leadership to a parental context, introducing the Educational Leadership for Parents framework that I have developed as a training program and will draw on here.

This chapter is divided into three sections:

- Educational Leadership for Parents: Principle and Practice
- Educational Leadership for Parents: Encouragement
- Educational Leadership for Professionals: Educators, Administrators, and Related Providers

Educational Leadership Defined

According to American University's School of Education description, educational leadership is an educational system approach that unites everyone under a common goal and a core set of values. The University of South Dakota describes educational leaders as scholar-practitioners who can solve complex problems of practice, with skills such as evidence-based research and critical thinking. Educational leadership is a graduate-level discipline where at both universities and other educational settings, transformational leadership is valued. Administrators such as district superintendents, school principals, and special education directors are considered educational leaders having such skills and values. Teachers and staff can also operate as educational leaders.

Educational Leadership for Parents: Principle and Practice

The first principle of Educational Leadership for Parents is that parents are the primary teachers: Parents are teachers, appointed by the Creator to provide the tools and resources to rear their children. One significant resource is the schoolteacher, who is usually certified by the state or federal body, or approved by a community to teach students. Why not work together? Educational Leadership for Parents says that the parent sets the tone for collaboration and leverages the strengths of both the parent and the teacher and all additional resources the child needs to be successful in the parent-chosen educational environment.

One myth that some parents have about teaching their children is that a significant amount of experience is required to be a schoolteacher. While academic experience is valuable, the lack of experience does not have to impede learning. Actually, there is no correlation between teacher experience and achievement (Rand, 2010). Evidence shows that general education teachers with a few years of experience are more effective than new teachers and that teacher effectiveness plateaus around five years (The New Teacher Project, 2016).

Another myth about parents being educational leaders is that they must be smart and know math, writing, and reading. Have you ever heard Dr. Ben Carson tell the fascinating story of how, when in fifth grade, his mother could not read, yet demanded he and his brother read and write book reports? She even pretended that she was literate and graded their papers. Dr. Ben Carson became the world's greatest brain surgeon and U.S. Secretary of Housing and Urban Development.

I developed Educational Leadership for Parents in 2013 after reflecting on my experiences, the triumphs of the matriarchs before me, mothers of children with disabilities, and Black mothers particularly, who lacked awareness and resources. Essentially, I wanted to empower lay parents with the leadership mindset and the educational leadership discipline's insights to leverage their parental role as active leaders in the child's learning, regardless of where they are taught.

The three accountabilities within the Educational Leadership for Parents framework are to:

(I.) Leverage Education - Appreciating the value of education, and the various education models, systems and functions.

(II.) Demonstrate Leadership – Recognizing leadership skills and applications for various education situations and settings.

(III.) Educate Intentionally – Facilitating resources with contexts such as early learning and differentiation for special needs.

Educational Leadership for Parents is supported by seven competencies and practices:

1. **Accepting:** the parent's role as the primary teacher
2. **Envisioning:** parental teaching, learning values and vision
3. **Identifying:** parent abilities, skills, and knowledge needed
4. **Decision Making:** parental research and choices of the right connections, collaborations, and curriculum
5. **Planning:** parent design of relevant, strategic, celebratory, and supportive goals and tasks
6. **Monitoring:** parental observations, documentation, collaboration, and sense-making
7. **Adjusting:** parental modification and clarification of plans, and assessment of successes and opportunities

Educational Leadership for Parents: Encouragement

Educational Leadership for Parents helps parents, future parents, grandparents, counselors, and therapists to plan, navigate, participate, and fully advocate to get the most out of their home, public, or private school education. ELP encourages parents to regard their parental role as honorable and to command respect for their education decisions.

A parent's honorable role is to nurture their child's growth and development from birth to adulthood, and it is quite a responsibility. Nurturing the physical body with health and nutrition is commonly accepted as the most essential task while the weightier matters of nurturing the spirit and mind with wisdom and education are often omitted. This principle demands a conscious effort to lift the burdens that deficiencies in wisdom and education cause families and societies at large.

Educating children is even more difficult when parents are undereducated, unmotivated, or unavailable. As a result, parents often find it difficult to:

- recognize cognitive development stages or "sensitive periods" (and may fail to make the responses required);
- exercise patience through behavior changes;
- understand and support teacher or school requirements;
- sustain the energies and time to find appropriate solutions;
- and understand how to implement solutions for the ideal effectiveness and success.

The most satisfying outcomes are obtained by those parents who sustain the mental and physical energies required to regularly discover, plan, and partner in their child's education. Parents need to acknowledge that managing their child's education requires endurance and patience, two principles that are as needful as water and impossible to separate as wetness is from water. Parents attempting to apply one without the other subsequently become followers instead of partners (let alone leaders), and many lose strength and withdraw involvement altogether. A mindset based on the principles in Educational Leadership for Parents and practice will equip and inspire parents to make good choices with wisdom from experts and successful parents alike to light and navigate their child's education pathway. (Jackson, M. 2013)

An Educational Leadership for Parents Example: BSSN-2E Mother

Educational Leadership for Parents (ELP) inspires BSSN mothers to dig deep within themselves, dig into the presented practices, and dig out of the hole of frustration. ELP offers teachers and school staff examples of encouragement to share with BSSN parents, and validates existing leadership examples, like JC who encourages other parents. Following is the testimony of JC, a BSSN parent who has had some success and challenges in breaking through those barriers to be an educational leader for her child:

> *I see twice-exceptional (2E) students as nothing short of amazing! Their intake and processing of information, communication, and social disposition do not match with what is considered to be standard or normal. Instead, 2E students navigate a complex set of emotional, cognitive, social, and other challenges, and somehow, their intellectual prowess is abnormal in that it far exceeds what is considered to be standard.*
>
> *I am the parent of a 12-year-old African American male who is twice-exceptional. My son is not as attentive or as socially comfortable as his peers. He has attention-deficit hyperactivity disorder (ADHD) and Social Pragmatic Disorder, both diagnosed in fourth grade. Long before there was awareness and support in place, he was academically advanced, reading books in English and Spanish at age four, scoring in the ninetieth percentile for standardized mathematics tests and in the eightieth percentile in standardized reading tests.*
>
> *The most dominant challenge has been with teachers pointing out characteristics they perceive to be negative. The same teachers presented no observation or acknowledgment of my son's strengths and no holistic evaluation to make a more informed determination of his true challenges and the support he needed to improve his performance.*

From first grade, my son exhibited characteristics in school such as lack of focus, difficulty managing emotions, and social awkwardness. He was often quiet, did not distract other students, and was able to perform well academically, read above grade level, and scored exceptionally on standard exams. I would hear from his teacher about his inattentiveness, emotional responses, and some minor differences with other students, but I never received an offer for further assessment or support. I believe that because he did not cause trouble and he was meeting academic standards, his teachers did not find it prudent to assess him further.

As a committed parent, I decided to explore further on my own and would regularly report back to teachers and administrative staff, and I still never received offers of support from the school. Over the years, I performed web-based research on characteristics my son displayed. As a result of the research, I engaged a therapist, obtained a private educational assessment, hired an occupational therapist, and finally obtained a full neuropsychological assessment. I engaged his teachers and other administrative staff every step of the way. And never did I receive an offer for further assessment or other support. And to my surprise, I learned through my research that his school district had a published resource readily available for their teachers and staff to use as a tool for identifying and supporting 2E students. Yet no support at all was offered to my son, who showed many of the characteristics of a 2E student. And even after all the effort of private testing, 504, and IEP assessment meetings, we received some 504 accommodations but still no social-emotional support or academic curricula that nurture his intellectual ability. I even had a teacher tell me that she did not believe that my son was suited for the gifted and talented program.

And that is when I realized that I would never receive, without a fight, the level of support from within the school district that is needed for my son to excel. So, each school year, I roll up my sleeves and engage with teachers and administrators in the school, asking questions, making

recommendations, offering support, and following up for accountability on all parts. It is an uphill battle, where sometimes I win, and sometimes, I learn. But each day, month, quarter, and school year, I will continue to fight to the very end for my son and other students who learn and process differently than what is perceived as standard.
C. Janeè Caslin

Bold Educational Leadership for Parents Advice for BSSN Parents

I had the pleasure of interviewing veteran education leader and retired attorney, Brenda Wolff. Ms. Wolff is a parent of two adult children and a devoted grandmother. She offers these points of advice for BSSN parents:

1. She says that parents should "exercise parents' rights to freedom of information," by placing a request for data on their child's school from the school district office.
2. She offers that "parents can apply to be paraeducators or substitute teachers."

Working inside the school or alongside your own child is a bold ELP practice. Under the ELP accountability of *Educate Intentionally*, parents can facilitate resources for special needs contexts. Particularly when schools are being challenged by staffing issues, BSSN parents can offer human resources to help the child/student progress. The mother of my BSSN client referred her family friend to the district for one of many unfilled Paraeducator positions. The Dedicated Aide service, also known as 1:1 (one-to-one) in her IEP, was not being implemented because of the staffing shortage. The family friend was interviewed, screened, hired, and then assigned to be my client's Dedicated Aide.

Bold ELP: Parent Advocacy

Another bold ELP strategy is advocacy. Advocacy is asserting one's rights when services are being denied/withheld. The full description and recommendation for advocacy as a solution are explored in Chapter 9. I mention it here as a call to educational leadership for parents to consider how to assemble the tools to *access* advocacy. Parents have "shared many concerns about collaborating with educators," including fears and anxieties resulting from a lack of communication and trust, as well as negative perceptions of disabilities. The way a family may be made to feel, diverse languages, depth of communications, and perceptions about special education all differ across community groups.

The Government Accountability Office (GAO) identified several challenges that prevent parents of color and lower income from accessing their rights under IDEA. These challenges or barriers keep parents from getting help or using their own voice to advocate and get to resolution with the school system for their child's free and appropriate public education. When interviewed by K-12 Dive about the GAO's 2019 IDEA Dispute Resolution Report, Senator Patty Murray (D-Washington) said, "We need to look carefully at barriers preventing parents who are low-income or of color from advocating for their children, and then fix those problems" (GAO, 2019). The report identified key reasons why parents do not access legal services and legal representation.

Barriers or Reasons Why Black or Latinx Parents Do Not Access IDEA Rights:

1. *Costs for Service:* Even if reduced or based on household income, high costs are a barrier to retaining advocacy or legal representation.

2. *Stigma:* Obtaining diagnosis, language isolation, negative perception of disabilities, or the assumption of accuracy from the expert.

3. *Service Awareness:* Parents and Providers are not aware of services, and limited access to student records.

4. *Fear:* In collaborating with educators, retaliation from the school, or poor communication and trust.

5. *Time:* Inability to take time from work to attend or prepare for meetings and related activities.

The SEE US (Special Education Excellence for Underserved Students) initiative which makes advocacy free and accessible for BSSNs is attempting to remedy barriers one and three. Educators engaging in professional development training and treating parents as partners in the BSSN's education help to overcome barrier number four. The U.S. Department of Labor broadened the use of Family Medical Leave Act (FMLA), which is employment-protected unpaid time off from work, to include attendance at IEP meetings. So, BSSN parents can use FMLA through their employer to attend their BSSN's IEP meeting. This can help address barrier five above, but only if the parent works for an employer that qualifies for FMLA. My hope is that *Pour the Water* offers some relief to barrier number two.

Educational Leadership for Professionals

While parents are positioning themselves for appropriate participation, education and related professionals must do the same. This section begins with professional perspectives in the form of responses from the professional development course, *Identifying and Removing Obstacles from Black Students with Special Needs* (Jackson, 2021), and strategies to use educational leadership principles and professional development guidance to be substantial parts of the *Pour the Water: Transformative Solutions for Equity & Justice in Special Education* ecosystem.

Perspectives of School Staff

In 2021, I administered a survey as part of a training on racialized inequity at a pre-dominantly white institution (PWI), a model school for students with developmental disabilities and giftedness on the East Coast. Most participants were graduate degree-level White teachers and staff. One hundred staff and teachers were asked to identify their personal and professional dilemmas regarding Black students and special education. Here are some of their voices:

- *I always feel I am balancing my own "liberal white guilt" against my desire to challenge all of our students.*
  Staff, Teacher
- *I find that personally and professionally, as a White person, I am anxious about creating spaces for Black students— I wonder how I can do this best without alienation.*
  Teacher
- *As a Black teacher, I am constantly worried that I am mirroring "code-switching" to our Black students. Although it is necessary to code-switch in a PWI at times, I wonder if modeling my two identities is confusing or harmful to their future selves.*
  Teacher
- *After attending a PWI with White professors and staff I feel as though the education did not prepare me to be trauma-informed. The impact of racism on students is traumatic, and I do not feel ready to help in the ways I want to help. In addition to that: As a white femme-presenting person, I know my image is inherently violent, and sometimes I feel lost as to what to do.* **Classroom Facilitator**
- *The difficulty of addressing more subtle racism in a classroom in a constructive rather than just critical way. In my experience, direct criticism of any negative behavior, while much better than ignoring it, tends to teach students to hide it rather than change it. However, holistic constructive criticism of topics as complicated as racism generally requires explicit and specific preparation and careful wording. So, my dilemma is this: How can I address subtle racism (i.e., assuming a student's behavior or habits based on their race versus using the n-word) in a constructive, explicit, and specific way without letting the moment pass?*
  Teacher

- *I have encountered a number of occasions in which the behavior of Black students—generally young Black boys—is viewed by White teachers as problematic; perceived as 'acting out' behavior. There has been some disagreement between teachers and parents regarding whether the behaviors are the problem, or whether the teacher's preconceived notions of appropriate behaviors and responses to behaviors are discriminatory or biased against Black students with special needs. It has been difficult to know how to reconcile teacher classroom expectations and these behaviors in an anti-racist way that facilitates honest communication between teachers and parents.*
  Administrator
- *Finding ways to not be complicit in perpetuating White supremacy, particularly in the school setting, which does exactly that and worse for our Black students facing that and their learning differences...*
  Teacher
- *My main concern is that I don't have the freedom to speak as frankly about the truth of systemic issues without offending the ideology of parents.* **Teacher**
- *Perceptions and biases of non-Black administrators and teachers towards Black students (and teachers).*
  Teacher
- *" Black and Brown students not having previously been diagnosed or treated for learning issues and attention issues.*
  School Nurse
- *Am I aware of and addressing all issues related to Black students so that they are supported in the way they want and need?*
  Related Service Professional
- *I continuously go back to Lisa Delpit's Other People's Children and address how I interact with students of color, how upbringing forms the lens through which we see, and being conscious of how that comes out.*
  Teacher and Administrator

Recognizing and then sharing personal and professional dilemmas is a vulnerable, yet valuable exercise. Facilitating deeper reflections and related activities in the professional development process gives educators the encouragement they need to apply learned practices. With such tools, they can continue working toward equity for BSSNs.

The Education Team

Professionals in the list below are all key participants, in and out of the school, who participate in the successes of BSSNs or in the failure that is the school-to-prison/deportation/death pipeline:

- Administrators
- Advocates
- Attorneys
- Counselors
- Parents
- Physicians
- Psychologists
- Specialists
- Teacher-General Ed
- Teacher-Special Ed
- Therapists

Individualized Education Plan (IEP) Team

The IEP team is the decision-making body of **school-based professionals** who determine identification (or eligibility), interventions, and placement. This team can be pretty intimidating to parents, particularly when parents need clarification on the roles, positions, and power each holds. Demystifying the EMT (Education Management Team) and IEP teams can help. The school psychologist is this team's most influential member, the one who holds the data about the student's intelligence and academic functioning. While no one member holds a single authority, members tend to yield to the findings of the school psychologist to determine educational disability. The school psychologists' and teachers' conclusions or recommendations can be limited by implicit or explicit bias, insufficient data, or intimidation by outside/medical psychologists. The key players on the IEP team and their roles are highlighted below.

Administrators

Administrators may not have many direct observations of the BSSN to add to educational disability determination. However, they can significantly influence the BSSN's IEP process by mitigating bias, examining data, and facilitating the balance of perspectives. Administrators (with the case manager) might give close attention to the following to influence special education equity for BSSNs:

- Facilitate appropriate stakeholders' participation in IEP and 504 process.
- Provide cultural competency, disability-specific, and trauma-informed professional development training, coaching, and supervision.
- Ensure teacher quality, quantity, and representation.
- Review reports and forms for biased language (e.g., "he is aggressive") and cultural competence.
- Ensure parent support.
- Support teacher instruction of critical thinking and leadership.

Administrators can educate all teachers on bias. We tend to be acutely aware of our perceptions of others. We can sense confidence through the style of dress. We can hear ethnicity through language accents. We can see racial constructs through skin tone. Implicit biases are expected and part of our life experiences, as described in the works of the Kirwan Institute's Study of Race and Ethnicity at Ohio State University. The problem comes when we allow our bias to rule in decision-making. As we have seen, multiple research studies demonstrate that a child's race and ethnicity are significantly related to the probability of being inappropriately identified as disabled.

Counselors

School counselors are generally relegated to academic credit guidance and social-emotional training. The function is one of the most underutilized and under-resourced school positions. The American Counseling Association (ACA) Advocacy Competencies describe necessary general counselor skills, knowledge, and behavior that can be implemented to address systemic barriers and issues facing students, clients, client groups, or whole populations (hereafter, clients and client groups are inclusive of students and student groups) (House & Toporek, 2022). Encourage counselors to identify and address systemic issues more broadly. The Advocacy Competencies focused on the role of counselors as advocates working with or on behalf of their clients who were struggling with systemic barriers. Counselors can advocate on behalf of clients/children/students in various settings. ACA Competency Clusters include direct interventions, environmental interventions, school community, and system leadership. The following list highlights the ACA Advocacy Competencies:

- Identify strengths and resources of clients and students.

- Identify the social, political, economic, and cultural factors that affect the client/student.

- Recognize the significance of the counselor's own cultural background and sociopolitical position in relation to power, privilege, and oppression and in relation to the client or client communities.

- Recognize signs indicating that an individual's behaviors and concerns reflect responses to systemic or internalized oppression.

- At an appropriate developmental level and cultural perspective, help the individual identify the external barriers that affect his, her or their development.

- Share resources and tools that are appropriate for the client/student's developmental level and issue.

- Train students and clients in self-advocacy skills.

- Help students and clients develop self-advocacy action plans.

- Assist students and clients in carrying out action plans.

- Identify barriers to the well-being of clients and students with attention to issues facing vulnerable groups.

- Recognize the significance of the counselor's own cultural background and sociopolitical position in relation to power, privilege, and oppression and in relation to the client or client communities.

- Identify potential allies for confronting the barriers, including those within the organization as well as those who have cultural expertise relevant to the client's issue.

- Develop an initial plan of action for confronting these barriers in consultation with the client and ensuring the plan is consistent with the client's goals.

- Communicate the plan with the client, including rationale and possible outcomes of advocacy.

- Negotiate relevant services and education systems on behalf of clients and students.
- Help clients and students gain access and create a plan to sustain needed resources and support.
- Carry out the plan of action and reflect/evaluate the effectiveness of advocacy efforts.

Psychologists

School psychologists are generally the leading voice on behavior and disability identification. The practice of psychology includes consultation, assessment/evaluation, therapy, research, training, and advocacy. Psychologists are a diverse community that includes independent practitioners and institutional practitioners in multidisciplinary settings, including schools, health care facilities, university counseling centers, community mental health centers, state and federal prisons, and military services.

Teachers

Early childhood and elementary teachers are especially precious to a child with special needs. Unfortunately, the promise, progress, and practices students with special needs experience in early intervention and pre-K are simply not prolonged afterward. As students complete kindergarten, first grade, second grade, and third grade, we often see lessening of progress for BSSNs. Parents and advocates observe a lack of quality of care, infidelity of special education services, and limitations in general education's instructional flexibility, among other systemic shortcomings that begin to impact the BSSN. BSSN students in particular typically fare far worse than their WSSN peers, given the extensive systemic impacts and other variables, adding another layer of frustration for BSSN teachers and parents. Developing teacher qualities in compassion, advocacy, and bias can make a difference.

Teacher quality in compassion can make a difference. As much as teacher preparation programs teach instructional skills, they must equally employ empathy. Empathy will motivate the teacher to develop new skills, keep consistent communications with BSSN parents, apply behavior-nurturing strategies, and be equitable in applying interventions and referrals for BSSNs.

The referring classroom teacher influences team decision-making as the first-line observer of academic tasks, social interactions, and adaptive functioning. Advocacy skills should also be a part of every teacher's skillset. The teacher's ability to use data, observations, communication, collaboration, and conviction all serve the best interest of the BSSN. When teachers advocate for BSSNs, they accept accountability for the success of the BSSN.

Teacher Representation

Second, to a parent, there is nothing else like a teacher's love. High-quality teachers across all racial groups spend their days and nights planning and worrying about the students they serve. Research shows that this love translates better in classrooms where the teachers and students are of the same race. (Strive Together 2021) reports,

> *If you have a teacher of your race, you are more likely to receive fairer grades and discipline as well as an increased likelihood of graduating and going to college. Bright Futures used local data to illustrate the disparity in student and teacher representation in school districts. This is one of the data points that led to a greater focus on teacher pathways.*

Research has consistently shown the positive effects of having a teacher of the same race on various student outcomes. However, the literature has yet to examine how racial match affects everyday interactions within classrooms. Research by Battey et al., 2018, addresses this underexplored area by documenting relational interactions in classrooms to find one mechanism that could produce racialized effects on learning. Using a dataset from a study of twenty-five mathematics classrooms across predominantly White and Black U.S. middle schools, they examine the quality of relational interactions when teachers and students are racially matched and mismatched and the effects on student achievement in mathematics. Their analysis shows how various dimensions of relational interactions significantly predict increases and decreases in achievement due to racial match.

So, with this burgeoning data, one may continue to pose the question, was the desegregation of schools productive? Were the Hyde County anti-desegregation activists predicting system failure? While more research will likely emerge on same-race teaching as the 70th Anniversary of Brown vs. Board of Education approaches, some in the field already report seeing differential treatment in the classrooms and the discussions around same-race teachers are growing.

Cultural Competence

Cultural competence is awareness of one's own cultural identity and views about differences and the ability to learn about and build on the varying cultural and community norms of others (NEA, n.d.).

When individuals (or organizations) are culturally competent, they acknowledge and incorporate at all levels the importance of culture, the assessment of cross-cultural relations, the expansion of cultural knowledge, and the adaptation of services to meet cultural development needs (Cross et al., 1989).

While cultural identity is commonly displayed outwardly through clothing, music, dance, or food, it also exists in the display of behaviors, word choice, and desires. Transformative leadership can help foster cultural identity development in these less obvious areas of BSSN culture that often have a significant impact on the goals and strategies for academic and social success. Behaviors, word choice, and desires are often norms formed at home or in the community, sometimes outside of school.

Culturally Responsive Teaching

Dr. Geneva Gay (2010) defines culturally responsive teaching as "Using the cultural characteristics, experiences, and perspectives of ethnically diverse students as conduits for teaching them more effectively" (p. 31). Culturally responsive teachers include the presence of BSSN's cultural contexts as a means of making communicating curriculum more effective. They also consider the continual exploration of culture, particularly given some family's cultural reexaminations and quests to revitalize their past culture (known as cultural revitalization). BSSNs who have social and cognitive limitations, for example will need support as they adapt to application of culture connected to academic expectations. We also need culturally competent assessors.

Culturally Responsive Curriculum

A culturally responsive curriculum (a) ensures that all students are interested and engaged; (b) connects to what culturally different students want to learn, (c) presents a balanced, comprehensive, and multidimensional view of the topic, issue, or event; (d) presents multiple viewpoints; and addresses stereotypes, distortions, and omissions (Banks, 2008). As evidenced by the numerous clarifications in the book, *Lies My Teacher Told Me* by the late Professor and Racial Activist James Loewen, we owe it to our students to examine curriculum truths of history and culture. In her book, *Culturally Responsive Teaching*, Dr. Geneva Gay states that "Content about the histories, heritages, contributions, perspectives, and experiences of different ethnic groups and individuals, taught in diverse ways, is essential to culturally responsive teaching" (p. 127, 2010).

In the 1980s retired special educator and pioneer Dr. Robert Felton hypothesized that Bowen theory could aid BSSNs. Dr. Felton believed that if BSSNs knew more about their personal multigenerational history, they would do better in school. He thought that "If the families and parents were learning about their history, then the children would also be engaged." Dr. Murray Bowen was a psychiatrist whose life work was a family systems theory that, among other things, sought to understand the family, rather than the individual, as an emotional unit. His theory also considers understanding one's multigenerational family emotional process as key in understanding one's functioning and health. Bowen theory, a science of human behavior, has concepts that are applicable for problem-solving among families, communities, and organizations. Dr. Felton petitioned his school district leadership to start a program that would support looking at family history together with the family. However, his supervisors at the time would not allow him to implement the program, suggesting it was "too controversial."

Chapter Activity for Educational Professionals

Professional Development Workshop

Educators and related professionals can use the workshop prompt detailed below to introduce equity for Black students with special needs.

Title: Introduction to Identifying and Removing Obstacles for Black Students with Special Needs

Audience: Educators (teachers, staff, and administrators) and Professionals inexperienced in producing high-quality outcomes for BSSNs.

Duration: 90 minutes per topic

Description: Through an interactive and energetic video conference, teachers and staff will learn the relationship between racism and special education, exploring the factors that create and make obstacles impassable for Black students with special needs. High school regression, the school-to-prison pipeline, and unemployment outcomes are almost double the rate for Black students with special needs than White students and higher than for Latino and Indigenous students, the other two educationally underserved populations. Responsible awareness of special education, White supremacy, fragility and allyship, historical oppression from slavery and bias, and parental disempowerment will be explored through lecture and discussion.

Strategy: Data and examples from *Pour the Water: Transformative Solutions for Equity & Justice in Special Education* will be selected based on team interests and needs and compiled for participants. Best practices from effective educators will be provided for participants. Participants will partner to identify one tool or strategy to address each target (e.g. racial bias) within the participant's teaching or support role that will improve student learning experiences and outcomes. Participants will report out highlights after a set time (ex., 20 min). Workshop activities include an alumni panel, staff discussions, grade-level groupings, questions for discussion, and reflections. Discussions include evaluating students based on value and merit rather than race, culture, or socioeconomic status; and the losses and gains when Black students with special needs attend a predominately White school.

Outcomes: Upon completion of this workshop, participants will be able to:

- Recognize teacher and staff responsibility to identify and remove obstacles for Black students with special needs.

- Identify successful transitions and school-based strategies for including Black students in a predominately or historically White populated school or community.

- Solve an ethical dilemma or scenario related to bias and systemic racism.

Chapter 7

Education Equity Through Prioritization and Desire: Nine Passionate Priorities

GOAL

Given the prioritization of on grade-level reading, self-directed learning, early intervention, inclusion, and data disaggregation, BSSNs will receive equitable education for their gifts, differences, or disabilities by (e.g., June 2026), as measured by improvement in academic reading scores, transition plan engagement, intervention success by eight years of age, and separate data reporting for Black descendants of emancipated slaves, as tracked on record.

CHAPTER INTRODUCTION

The priority of equity in the education of BSSNs as an act of justice is outlined in this chapter. This chapter examines why the prioritization in an exclusive way of Black students is necessary to fulfill education equity. Key priorities, addressing issues that educators find perplexing, and that BSSNs and their families are persistently plagued by, are presented. Readers will be able to gauge their desire for change and question their capacity to deliver.

Is the Broad Approach Effective?

While the Biden Administration signed executive orders on action to promote racial justice and equity, the orders are quite broad. The orders promote and define equity as

> ...the consistent and systematic fair, just, and impartial treatment of all individuals, including individuals who belong to underserved communities that have been denied such treatment, such as Black, Latino, and Indigenous and Native American persons, Asian Americans and Pacific Islanders and other persons of color; members of religious minorities; lesbian, gay, bisexual, transgender, and queer (LGBTQ+) persons; persons with disabilities; persons who live in rural areas; and persons otherwise adversely affected by persistent poverty or inequality. (The White House)

Under the guise of equity for one group or purpose, the inclusive approach actually waters down any meaningful aid, effectively negating the help for the target group. This has historically been the case for Blacks in America and the reason why transformation is impossible. Passive for everyone nullifies the help for the targeted one.

On this principle, words by Ta-Nehisi Coates from his, *We Were Eight Years in Power: An American Tragedy* come to mind: "Compassion and pragmatism make for ambiguous policy" (T. Coates, 2017). Let us say there are three teams with a goal of all three getting 10 points. One team is at -12 points, another at -7 points, and the other at +3 points. Mathematics tells us that the -12 team would need 22 points, the -7 team would need 17, and the +3 team would need 7 points. Providing the team with 22 points and the other group with only 7 points might not seem fair or equal, but it is equitable. Before we can get to equality, we have to get to equity.

Racial equity is "a process of eliminating racial disparities and improving outcomes for everyone. It is the intentional and continuous practice of changing policies, practices, systems, and structures by prioritizing measurable change in the lives of people of color" (Government Alliance on Race and Equity). While we can learn about racial equity from this definition, when you include "people of color" or "everyone" it is not equity and has limited effectiveness. As *P.A.R.E.N.T.S. Life Skills,*

Literacy, & Leadership Framework for Social Change Co-Author, Kirk Jackson commented about such a practice, "It is actually a ruse, to abuse, and everyone is confused as to why the Blacks always lose."

Prioritizing Black Students with Special Needs is an Act of Justice, and Emphasizing Priorities Will Yield Education Equity

BSSNs must be prioritized for all the reasons outlined in this book, and for the millions of unnamed souls lost to slavery, incarceration, and murder in America, coupled with the billions of unearned dollars. I have revealed several realities and root causes of injustice and made plain critical impacts and solutions for equity. Your opportunity is to see and accept this justification for prioritization, to create change in practices, culture, resources, and systems.

BSSN Priorities

We must desire "D.E.S.I.R.R.R.R.E." Education Equity for BSSNs through the following priorities:

1. *D*ata through disclosure and disaggregation *"Prioritize Data Discovery for BSSNs"*
2. *E*xpectations raised in gifted identification and in generating cultures of learning: *"Prioritize Higher Expectations for BSSNs"*
3. *S*elf-Direction, through self-directed learning: *"Prioritize Self-Direction for BSSNs"*
4. *I*nclusion through belonging, in school, community, and programs: *"Prioritize Inclusion for BSSNs"*
5. *R*eading, through scientific, evidence-based methodologies and remediation: *"Prioritize Reading for BSSNs"*
6. *R*emediation, through targeted training and supports. *"Prioritize Remediation for BSSNs"*

7. **R**eset for resilience and emotional care in calming spaces and residential placements: *"Prioritize Resetting for BSSNs"*

8. **R**espite and relief for parents of BSSN: *"Prioritize Respite for BSSN Parents"*

9. **E**arly intervention in early childhood education: *"Prioritize Early Intervention for BSSNs*

Educational Equity: What Is It?

According to the Child Opportunity Index, Black children are between six and nine times more likely than white children to live in areas of concentrated poverty. (diversitydatakids.org, 2020) The Federal Government has policies and research to support equity. Part A (Title I) of the Elementary and Secondary Education Act, as amended by the Every Student Succeeds Act (ESSA), provides financial assistance to Local Educational Agencies (LEAs) and schools with high numbers or high percentages of children from low-income families to help ensure that all children meet challenging state academic standards. In 2013, The Equity and Excellence Commission examined the disparities in meaningful educational opportunities that give rise to the achievement gap, focusing on systems of finance, and recommended ways in which federal policies could address such disparities. My Brother's Keeper for example, connects young people to mentoring, support networks, and the skills they need to find a good job or go to college and work their way into the middle class.

What is Desire?

Desire must be prevalent in order to make a substantive difference. My experiences as a college-level student-athlete, top-tier sales rep, several-time natural birthing conqueror, and even being an expert special education advocate taught me that the desire for achievement is fortified by dedication to discipline and strategy for targeted and tracked goals. Starting each of these five SEE US solutions chapters, a goal is written in the format of an IEP goal, using the SMART framework: Specific, Measurable, Attainable, Relevant, and Time-bound.

I hope that together we seek to meet these desired outcomes. Desire is not passive nor satisfied with sufficiency; it is the dedication to efficient strategies and supports for success. Love will serve as our guiding principle to win, and we must recognize that our competition is poverty, including poverty of the mind and spirit that only a change in mindset, education, and knowledge will defeat.

A great illustration of modern-time desire can be found in two words: Michael (and) Jordan. The name Michael (the name of the biblical archangel of war) and Jordan (the last river crossing of the Hebrews before entering the promised land) signifies a calling to be great. Michael Jordan's mother expected it, his teammates and coaches felt it, and the endorser suitors and fans wanted a piece of it.: the desire to win, the passion, emotion, and intense focus to finish first. He was not always the top basketball player; he was placed on the J.V. team for further development. Michael Jordan grew up around racism— being called the N-word— and was even suspended from school for his response to it. Desire is what he used to overcome obstacles. As he said in the documentary, The Last Dance, "my mentality was to go out and win at any costs" and he did.

It is okay to use great athletes, artists, scientists, and entrepreneurs as examples of passion as long as we teach our children how to generalize. Generalization is to take characteristics from one situation and apply them to another. Generalization is not an automatic skill; it has to be taught. BSSNs with autism struggle immensely with generalization. Interventions such as social stories and speech services to develop pragmatic language skills are invaluable. BSSNs can benefit from social studies and history curricula for examples of how people relate and function within and across societies.

Achievement barriers can be impassable obstacles to desiring something one cannot see. Let us use the following BSSN DESIRRRRE practices to reveal the vision for BSSN Education Equity.

DESIRRRRE Education Equity for BSSNs

D-DATA – Prioritize Data Discovery for BSSNs

Having accurate data and understanding the meanings of the data is necessary for evaluating solutions. Data gathering and reporting must be ethical and careful. Dr. Claud Anderson admonishes that utilizing data for a specific agenda or to further a cause is not uncommon and needs to be administered appropriately. We are all familiar with horrible scenarios like the Tuskegee torture and that the practice of modern gynecology originated in the dismantling of Black women's wombs for the sake of science. Now, with the Institutional Review Board (IRB), research has some oversight.

Ethics & Responsibility

Data ought to be just as ethically and carefully communicated. Simple data soundbites through media channels can be disheartening without context or guidance. For example, the MAP data published in 2022 in Baltimore, Maryland, showed that zero students in twenty-three schools were proficient in math (for which first Black Governor of Maryland, Wes Moore says he expects accountability), created valid curiosity and concern among parents and the community. When reviewing the education data, these were helpful perspectives to consider: What actual school year(s) does the data include? What were the prior year's scores, trends and patterns? How did the pandemic influence the scores? How does the class/school/district compare to other classes/schools/ districts? The most important question: Who is most impacted and why?

Data on poverty for example, can provide some answers, but not all. Data reporting on percentages of poverty and percentages are useful but not always clear because poverty categories are aggregated (Sen, 1983). As Ta-Nehisi Coates points out in, *When We Were Eight Years in Power,* "Black poverty and White poverty are not the same" (Coates, 2017). He clarifies that the poverty gaps are not the same; there is an *injury gap* and an *achievement gap.* Education focuses on achievement, but doing more in education won't close the injury gap. Many black students are starting from a place of disadvantage, and this must be addressed before the achievement gap can be closed.

The Achievement Gap is rooted in deficit thinking, for it places the onus of addressing educational disparities on the very students who experience inequities because it suggests that students are failing to achieve. The term equity gap, on the other hand, evokes the notion that institutions are responsible for creating equity for students. Institutional leaders and practitioners might consider their use of deficit-minded language when discussing equity changes and data analysis. We want to avoid language that communicates the expectation that (BSSNs) are expected to create equity for themselves re

The Data Count for Descendants of US Chattel Slavery

The Missouri Compromise of 1820 allowed Black slaves to be counted as part of the human population. You may recall that the:

> *…Three-fifths provision applied only to Blacks. It did not apply to indentured servants, White women, children, native Indians, Asians, Hispanics or any group included in today's fabricated classes of minorities. (Anderson, 2018)*

Dr. Anderson continues that,

> *The Electoral College system still counts on Black bodies to win seats but avoids representing Black interests in race matters and seldom provide Blacks with tangible benefits to improve their quality of life. (Anderson, 2018)*

Stakeholders must continue exploring decolonization in data discoveries and asking questions surrounding the equitable allocation of resources.

The U.S. Census Bureau collects race data in accordance with guidelines provided by the U.S. Office of Management and Budget (OMB), and these data are based on self-identification (US Census.gov). The racial categories included in the census questionnaire generally reflect a social definition of race recognized in this country, and not an attempt to define race biologically, anthropologically, or genetically. Descendants of emancipated slaves and current or multigenerational immigrants from Africa and the West Indies are defined by the U.S. census as black racial groups of African origin, also known as "Black." It defines "White" as people in Europe, the Middle East, or North Africa; "American Indian or Alaska Native" as people of North, South, and Central America; "Asian" as people from Japan, China, and India; and "Native Hawaiian." Selections are based upon self-identification and more than one category can be selected for persons claiming two or more races (Census.gov).

You can see that the racialized categorization "Black" attempts to denote similarity by skin tone, not by the unique characteristics of lived experiences or cultural identities. It does not reflect the unique experiences of a set of people with a horrific, multi-century American experience of chattel slavery and a post-Emancipation reality of racial discrimination. The collective "Black" does not extract the unique experiences of a set of people who have lived with the trauma of slavery and the devastating loss of riches in language and peculiarity. Oppressed for nearly 14 generations, anti-Black policies and practices have continued to adversely impact Freedman Blacks in the forms of addiction, poverty, and the school-to-prison pipeline. Against all odds, they have maintained the resilience and intelligence to retain community and revitalize culture. The distinction between descendants of chattel slavery and recent immigrant Africans should be distinguished.

According to American Descendants of Slavery (ADOS), "Ours is an experience defined by the unique, shared cost of multigenerational plunder." While ADOS's mission is focused on reparations, it also "insists upon a specific group designation." DAS (Descendants of Slaves) is also proposed as a Census category, essentially for a classification separate from immigrant Africans and other Blacks. The DAS petition would create a new citizenship category where DAS is "properly recognized" and resources are "properly designated."

DAS (Descendants of American Slaves) describe the class as "uniquely American." DAS declare its class as the offspring of those born into American slavery whose culture was not acknowledged and abandoned and is still dealing with the ramifications of American Slavery. Cited on the DAS website,

> *We, Descendants of American Slaves, believe in the necessity of claiming our birthright & inheritance to establish the Kingdom of God that ensures the (economic) empowerment of our families, communities, and the world for the commonwealth of all humanity.*

ADOS says that "any future studies or data collection by the U.S. government must disaggregate ADOS from the rest of the American population so that the specific needs of ADOS communities can be accurately quantified and addressed by targeted policies and investments." To be clear, multigenerational Black immigrants have suffered at the hand of systemic racism from colonization and slavery, too, just not at the same scope and magnitude. Prioritizing education equity for one group is a difficult decision, but one that the specific nation of Blacks requires. DAS4ESJ (Descendants of Slaves for Equity and Social Justice) believes in system change, as, "…long-term solutions that spread economic opportunity, power, and justice to every person."

Education data commonly compares and contrasts Black, Indigenous, Latinx, White, and Asian students. In most data samples, Asian, and Indigenous are the most underrepresented. Which categories do you notice? Why? Is the propaganda that Asians are the "model" minority a myth or truth? We know that Asian students with learning disabilities perform higher than black students with disabilities. We also know that the "Asian" category is aggregated with Chinese, Korean, Japanese, or Vietnamese. How is it possible to assume that this overcategorization can provide any insight into why or how the differences and similarities exist in disability student representation? One thing I remember from my undergraduate minor in Asian Studies was that all Asians are not alike, nor do they appreciate being generalized as being or having the same culture, experiences, and perspectives.

Informally, the labels "Brown" (non-Black and non-White), and "BIPOC" (Black, Indigenous, and People of Color) have emerged as alternatives to the census classifications. Given our desire to be intentional toward a target group and issue, let us be specific:

> *The Black population most impacted by systemic racism are descendants of the U.S. form of chattel slavery (a multigenerational bondage of monstrous brutality), and the Great Migration, who suffer today from its traumatic effects, systemic racism, oppression (unjust or cruel exercise of authority or power) and inequities in societal resources, particularly special education. (Jackson, M. 2020)*

How is Holistic Data Discerned?

Respect for group identity can be realized through holistic data discernment. Disaggregated data and related funding for educational resources is an exclusionary methodology and it is necessary to identify and address the root causes and solutions. However, there are times when disaggregated data discovery is necessary; this crisis of significant disproportionality and the school-to-prison pipeline is that time.

There are occasions when the special education gold standard of inclusion in the general education setting is not best for the BSSN. The BSSN would not be able to have his/her individualized education plan met in the inclusive setting and therefore needs to be educated in a school environment exclusive from the rest of his/her typically developing peers. When an MRE (more restrictive environment) is necessary to make meaningful progress, I let parents know that it does not have to be the final placement. BSSNs change developmentally and academically, and an appropriately facilitated IEP process will evaluate the decision annually and completely, with data breakdowns. BSSNs would receive resources specific to their needs with disaggregated data.

Interview with Brenda Wolff, JD

Retired educator and EEOC attorney, and past president of the Montgomery County Board of Education, Dr, Wolff has also served as the chair of the Negro Council of Women and was recognized as one of Maryland's Top 100 Women for her leadership, service and mentoring.

As part of my interview with this veteran educational leader, I asked her about the discipline disparity. She said, "Black people were always treated the worst." She told me about how she participated in departmental compliance reviews in the 1990s where disproportionality pointed to discipline as the cause of overrepresentation. The education districts reached a settlement where the resolution included reporting and training.

Long before her recent role as school board president, in 1999 she started a girl's mentoring program at Blake High School in Montgomery County, Maryland. The issue at the school for the Black girls then was disparate, over-discipline for the same infractions committed by White girls. For example, she said that for wearing a similar or same obscene outfit, the Black girl would experience body shaming and discipline, whereas the White girl would not. Black girls are mischaracterized as defiant and oversexualized (The Education Trust, 2020). In *Girlhood Interrupted: The Erasure of Black Girls' Childhood*, introduced the concept of adultification, where Black girls are "viewed as more adult and less innocent than their White peers" and "influence disproportionate exclusionary outcomes". (Georgetown Law Center on Poverty and Inequality, 2017)

Ms. Wolff says that compared to the late 90's, "discipline numbers may not be as bad as people think; the data has to be collected in the right way." Maryland has an example we can use regarding school discipline and data collection. Maryland says that "high-suspending" includes an elementary school that suspends 10% or more of its students in each subgroup, and a secondary school that suspends 25% or more of its students in each subgroup, disaggregated by race, ethnicity, disability status, and English language proficiency. The Maryland General Assembly House Bill 23 Ways and Means, Education, Health, and Environmental Affairs said that, effective July 1, 2022:

> *This bill requires the Maryland State Department of Education (MSDE) to make available, as a data download on its website, disaggregated discipline-related data at the State, local school system, and school levels. For all publicly available data, MSDE must include disaggregated data related to any disproportional disciplinary practices of a local school system or public school, as specified, and annually report the data to the Governor and the General Assembly. MSDE must report the disproportionality data for any school identified as "high-suspending" as specified and include alternative schools and programs and public separate day schools in any calculation of disproportionality data. (Maryland General Assembly)*

The StriveTogether community consortium in Kentucky recognized that a collection of factors, not only one, is necessary to realize change. Its mission is to make a collective impact, per community. StriveTogether values disaggregated data for strategic decisions.

> *"Our partnership had been working on disaggregating data, closing equity gaps and changing systems to some degree since our inception," Applegate said. "We disaggregated twenty-one measures by race, ethnicity, gender, language, disability, and socioeconomic, foster and housing status. Across nearly*

every indicator, the largest equity gap was race and ethnicity. And this was true when we looked at race and ethnicity combined with other identities. Racial equity gaps were still the largest, even among kids of the same socio-economic status." (Applegate, 2021)

Disaggregated Data Discovery Primer Questions

Deciding what to look for is a key principle of using data. BSSN Stakeholders can consider the following questions as they plan data discovery.

- What portion of BSSNs has an emotional disability due to a traumatic event vs. unexplained causation or genetic history?

- What portion of Black students who exhibit antisocial behavior have a medical condition, disability, or giftedness?

- What portion of BSSNs with autism receiving IEP-based psychological services are making progress on social-emotional and pragmatic language goals?

- What proportion of BSSNs who read two or more grades below level have progressed through tiers one, two and/or three responses to intervention?

Being equity-minded involves examining data disaggregated by race, noticing racial inequities in outcomes, and making sense of that data in critical ways. (Bensimon 2007; Bensimon and Malcolm 2012; Dowed and Bensimon 2015; Malcolm Picquet-Bensimon 2017). Equity can also be seen as "parity and representation, and outcomes for racially minoritized groups" (Bensimon, 2007; Bensimon & Malcolm, 2012) using and communicating data to advance equity. The goal of the equity parity standard is that all racial slash ethnic groups achieve an outcome rate equal to that of the highest performing group" (McNair et al., 2020).

To confirm the existence of inequities, data must be disaggregated by race, ethnicity, gender and disability, socioeconomic status, culture and region. Regarding the Black "race," the data must further be disaggregated by the participants' experiences. The root causes of inequities vary from subgroup to subgroup and across socioeconomic status, sex, and parent level of educational attainment. While generalizations can be made, they should not be the standard. For example, the experiences of immigrant Blacks from Africa to enslaved descendants in America are distinct. There is a distinctness to multigenerational Blacks as descendants of emancipated slaves with embedded traumas over hundreds of years who created a new culture and leveraged a formidable fight while living within the same entitled country and oppressive system. Racially minoritized students experience the classroom, socialization, and interactions with educators differently. Racially minoritized BSSNs are more negatively affected by special education decisions.

Data gathering alone is useless without proper sensemaking. While disaggregating data by race is a necessary step to advancing equity, it is also true that participants' contexts matter, and the broader social and historical context in which (an) institution is embedded should inform the specific racial and ethnic categories used (McNair, et al., 2020). After the data has been collected and analyzed, reporting and communication are important steps; data dashboards are a primary way to monitor and track data.

Sample Prompts to Guide Initial Discussions on Decisions to Disaggregate Data:

During planning sessions, teams will want to give consideration on how to construct data research or analysis. Prompts for the design of strategic data planning can help to discover factors important to the team and target group. Participants might use the following prompts in discussions:

- The persons or groups we will prioritize for goal setting are _____, because….

- We also need to collect additional data pertaining to _____ in order to understand the service gaps.
- We will seek to record patterns and trends related to _____, _____, and _____ based on observations of _____, _____, and ____.
- We will use the _____ systems and tools to track the data over the time period of _____ to ____.

Survey at the Source

I asked Dr. Doran Gresham, Assistant Professor of Special Education at The George Washington University, who specializes in teacher preparation for special education and is an expert in emotional disturbance, about the value of surveying around disproportionality and particularly to describe one he designed: the Gresham Survey.

Marcy: What is the Gresham Survey, started back in 2005, and why is it so important?

Doran: The greatest predictor of the future is the past, and the past is crystal clear in United States public education as it relates to the overidentification of Black males, particularly in restrictive classrooms for students with exceptionalities. For instance, educators, researchers, and policymakers have tracked the disproportionate representation of minorities in special education for 55 years, and we still haven't figured out ways to make the proportion of Black students in classrooms for students with special needs equal to those in general education. This isn't just a problem, it's a civil rights issue because once this particular group of students gets into these placements, not only do they not get out, but they become more likely to interact with officers, receive discipline referrals, and/or end up in the pre-K to prison pipeline. So, this survey was intended to go directly to the gatekeepers of this phenomenon, general education teachers, and determine what in the world is going on. After all, our students with exceptionalities are in general education before they are in special education, and they end up in these restrictive slower classrooms in part because we don't have enough specialists who can capture, inspire, and teach them. Essentially, what we might call compassionate coding is derailing the very population that it was intended to help in large part because of inherent biases and highly subjective disability categories.

Marcy: What metrics does the survey report on and from what key sources?

Doran: The survey was administered in a minority-majority school district in the D.C. area that oddly enough did not overrepresent elementary-aged black males in classrooms for students with emotional disabilities. The thought here was to go directly to people who might have cracked the code. For this research project, which was connected to my dissertation back in 2005, I created a 34-item Likert scale survey and it was administered to 163 elementary school general educators. From this number, 158 teachers responded to the survey, which was an unheard-of return rate of 97%. This group provided me with feedback about three central themes that impact this overrepresentation debate. They are as follows: school-related variables (e.g.: testing bias), teacher perception, and environmental factors, all of which play a part in this complex and persistent issue.

E-EXPECTATIONS- Prioritize Higher Expectations

Raising Expectations

Teachers and staff have a deep understanding that expectations impact student achievement. By not fostering high expectations for underserved and overserved students, prejudice prevails and becomes a platform for low expectations. For his 2000 NAACP presidential campaign address, former President Bush's speech writer, Michael Gerson, infused the phrase "soft bigotry of low expectations," to describe the internalization of mediocrity and poor performance among oppressed

Black children because of persistent racism and poverty. Biases associated with racial, ethnic, and disability identity make certain students more vulnerable to low expectations than others. In 2010, Montgomery County Public Schools in Maryland released *Equitable Classroom Practices,* a revised resource from 2006 with a call to consciousness from low expectations in the classroom for racialized disparities.

> *Though educators do not intend to communicate low expectations, the evidence that these societal beliefs have a tangible negative effect on the performance and achievement of students of color is well documented. Over time, low expectations hinder learning and negatively affect students' attitudes and motivation, resulting in self-fulfilling prophecies. Clearly, every educator must consciously and consistently demonstrate the specific, observable, and measurable behaviors and practices to all students regardless of their current academic performance if we are to eliminate persistent racial disparities in student achievement. (Montgomery County Public Schools, 2010)*

Establishing a culture for learning includes clear learning processes and expectations. One of the simplest reinforcement strategies for teachers is to provide attention and praise. This strategy is aimed at increasing the frequency of appropriate and adaptive behaviors and has been demonstrated to be an effective strategy for changing behavior. (Tresco, Lefler, Power, 2010). Provide appropriate standards and high expectations for all students. The absence of expectations and societal limitations does not allow us to explore our different learning and communication styles.

On any given day, there are dozens of reasons to recognize positive behaviors or even small successes. Each morning is a new opportunity to identify something special about your BSSN, including acknowledging the experiences that made him/her smart, courageous, and crafty. Design and refine the learning environment to facilitate and foster BSSN attributes that validate. This shapes the BSSN's expectation for representation and modeling. Posting culturally competent expectations in the front of the classroom (or at the beginning of a remote class) is a preventive strategy, particularly for BSSNs who are trauma-impacted. Routinely manage high expectations with reporting, recognition, responsibilities, and rewards depending on the individual needs of the BSSN.

Gifted Identification

Beyond Gifted Education author Scott Peters said that:

> *Nationally, students from African American, Latinx, and Native American families are underrepresented in gifted education by 43%, 30%, and 13% respectively (as of 2016); students with disabilities and who are still learning English are also underrepresented by roughly 75%. (2013)*

Parents and teachers should point out the potential in students as early as possible. Self-efficacy, academic self-confidence, and race consciousness are strategies to support BSSN with giftedness in the learning environment. Peters also said that the National Association for Gifted Children seeks to focus on "affirmative action policy, disseminating anti-racism information, overcoming racial and economic barriers, and changing the existing language to value equity and diversity."

Mathematics

Elevate the value of mathematical excellence. Help BSSNs feel like they belong as active learners, contributors, and models in math class. Studies conducted since 1989 have consistently shown that students are more likely to succeed in mathematics when they develop automaticity in basic math facts. Engineer Dr. Shamara Collins and retired teachers Dr. Marla Crawford, a special education specialist, and Dr. Darlene McCall, a science specialist, all support this point especially for Black students. Dr. McCall emphasizes the importance of algebra and the ability to problem-solve in preparation for scientific competency. Dr.

Collins says that effective math problem solving utilizes mental math and written form over a calculator tool as a valuable cognitive exercise.

Students who do not have math facts and procedures memorized are more likely to struggle with math problems because of working memory limits. According to the *International Electronic Journal of Mathematics Education*, the ability in mathematical reasoning and problem-solving is reinforced when there is an existing foundation of well-memorized math facts and procedures. (Hartman, 2023)

For certain BSSNs, mathematical memory can be a barrier if they have low working memory. Working memory is the ability to hold a micro-piece of information such as step or equation for use in the next part of the process. The article, *Should we Teach Children to Memorize the Multiplication Tables* cites,

> *Students who have not memorized math facts must temporarily interrupt their higher-level problem-solving processes to manually calculate (or type into a calculator) the product of 3 x 7. This is a diversion that pulls attention away from the actual problem, consumes space in working memory, and increases the risk of error (e.g., a student who counts to 22 while using a counting-up strategy to calculate 3 x 7). Proficiency in any field, not just mathematics, is built upon a foundation of automatized knowledge. (Hewitt & Sachdeva, 2023)*

S-SELF-DIRECTION-Prioritize Self-Direction

To support Self-Directed Learning, educators will need to raise expectations. Even though a BSSN might have a social or emotional disability, for example (like Nihcay), they likely have been raised in a home where self-determination is a core principle. Unsurprisingly, they experience this struggle between needing and receiving services. Self-directedness, or learner self-direction, refers to an individual's internal learning and growth process and the external influences experienced through instruction (Brockett & Hiemstra, 1991). Some BSSNs with social or emotional disabilities for example, may participate in taking the test but may not be motivated to perform to its standards.

Self-directed Learning

Self-directed learning is defined as a process of learning in which the individual establishes elements of control over their learning and characteristics of learners, including self-efficacy and motivation (Brockett & Hiemstra, 1991).

Self-direction skills are precursors to leadership skills. It is well regarded in the cultural scope of Blacks that leadership has always been an innate characteristic to be encouraged and taught. "Self-directed learning skills, also known as self-regulated learning skills, encompass three interrelated and mutually reinforcing areas (Institute of Education Sciences, 2021):

- **Affect**, which includes self-efficacy and the motivation to learn;
- **Strategic actions**, which include planning, goal setting, strategies to organize, code, and rehearse; and
- **Metacognition**, which includes self-monitoring, self-evaluating and self-correction.

Help students to connect language and social-emotional skills to soft skills that will be needed in the workplace. Self-regulation, communication and language skills are excellent discussion topics during the IEP process for BSSN. We saw the need for these skills in the emergency remote learning conundrum during the pandemic. Consider the performance of the BSSN and the need for self-efficacy goals to improve in these skill areas.

I-INCLUSION- Prioritize Inclusion for your BSSNs

Inclusion for BSSNs in the learning environment is impacted by the degree of belonging. In order to benefit from the inclusion, the BSSN needs to recognize a sense of belonging. The transformation for BSSNs is on a continuum of care, from fetus and infancy at home, to childhood and studenthood at school. From parents and teachers, BSSNs transform into independent young adults through guarantees of protection, provisions, nurture, and comforts. When that protection or nurture is absent, BSSNs can present antisocial behavior or learning disengagement in the classrooms based upon prior feelings of dissociation or not belonging. Ever heard a BSSN like Kevin in fourth grade say "Math isn't for me?" Where might that context have been shaped? We hope it was not in his teacher's third grade classroom where she marked red X's all over his classwork, or at home where Dad ignored school math nights but always made it for athletic game nights.

Parents and educators have an awesome responsibility to shape belonging since it is based on a simple social context of where one belongs. The practice of inclusion shapes the BSSN's awareness of belonging and is essential for the BSSN's success in secondary education and post-secondary outcomes. Here we meet two inclusion champions and opportunities where special education resources can be included.

Include BSSN in Schools—Example: Interview with Robert Felton, MA

Special Education Pioneer Robert "Bob" Felton retired in 2003 from special education and has served as a special education advocate for many years since then. He was a past supervisor of special education, a school principal, and the coordinator of special programs for students with mental retardation, as it was called then. Mr. Felton was a change agent and pioneer in the 1990s of the Home School model in Montgomery County, Maryland, for school inclusion of students with mild to moderate disabilities. School community-based programs in

Montgomery County started with a grant from the University of Maryland, to transition students from self-contained settings and started the home school model. This started nine community-based education classes, and now there are approximately sixty classes across the county.

Mr. Felton says that "All people with disabilities have a right to a full array of services in the communities." In his work in special education he wanted to teach the community how to relate to people with disabilities. He said that "people then had to learn how to relate to the students and incorporate practical life skills" training into the community activities to "help students to generalize," as in community-based instruction. People within communities protect a child more than when they are educated outside of the community; his motto is that "life begins in the community and should end in the community."

He said that the reasons people were apprehensive about inclusion "stemmed from their fear, ignorance, shame, and prejudice." He said that many White parents wanted their children to stay in the self-contained schools because they were ashamed of them. He pushed for students with mild intellectual disabilities and emotional disabilities to be transitioned from self-contained classes at various schools and for students with more moderate disabilities from special schools to integrate into classes at home/neighborhood schools closer to home. He said that often the more severe the child's disability, the further away from home the school seemed to be located.

His strategy was that funding could be better spent by placing the services where the child lives. By consolidating the services and resources into the schools, more teachers, for example, would be in a home school to serve students with special needs and disabilities. Principals supported the change to keep students in the home school; they could account for more staff and not need another program. He also developed team teaching training for co-taught instruction and other programmatic support. His conviction was that "special education is a set of services, not a place"; I would add that it is also not permanent.

It is well observed that students with disabilities do not fare well in long-term self-contained inappropriate placements. Their exposure and progress on graduation outcomes, social skills, and job readiness skills are wanting. For BSSNs, the impact of these inappropriate and irresponsible placements is devastating. Mr. Felton goes on to say:

> *The Supreme Court said that "separate but equal" did not work for people of color, and I believe that separate but equal does not work for people with disabilities. There is no right way to do the wrong thing. I have been called an "exclusionista" when advocating for people with disabilities. I believe people with disabilities are capable, complete human beings in their unique way, with equal rights. I believe that school systems across the nation have used special education programs as a way of promoting segregation of Black students by setting up self-contained classes and special education schools, especially for students classified as emotionally disturbed or intellectually disabled. (Robert Felton)*

Include BSSN in the Community

In *Adults with Developmental Disabilities: A Comprehensive Approach to Medical Care*, for the *American Family Physician Journal*, Dr. Kripke promotes accommodations and access for individuals with developmental disabilities. She writes that,

> *Regardless of functional limitations, with appropriate medical care, accommodations, and decision-making support, persons with developmental disabilities/ intellectual disabilities can live quality lives in their own homes and communities. Accommodations can include disability services, housing modifications, and adaptive equipment. (Kripke, 2018)*

Based on the Americans with Disabilities Act Title I Section 101 which has the following policy statement: "Disability is a natural part of the human experience that does not diminish the right of individuals with developmental disabilities to live independently, to exert control and choice over their own lives, and to fully participate in and contribute to their communities through full integration and inclusion in the economic, political, social, cultural, and educational mainstream of United States society."

School and community engagement activities can be geared toward individuals' various likes and preferences, which may differ among individuals. Karla Nabors has been a longtime, highly decorated defender of young adults with disabilities for over thirty years and is a champion for inclusion. She leads the Montgomery College Developmental Education (DE) program, whose mission is to: "Empower individuals to live, learn, work, and participate in the social fabric of our community. We believe, given the opportunity and proper support, all individuals can achieve academic success, successful careers, and personal growth."

I became an admirer of Karla's passion in 2007 as I created the Developmental Driver Education (DDE) program. I had observed that certain students with social and cognitive limitations were not completing the driver education program. As any good programmer would do, I discovered the relevant data and programmed relevant solutions. Observing Karla's outstanding student and family service helped me to deliver quality experiences and develop professionally in disability education. Forming connections between DE and DDE programs for students to expand learning opportunities was special,

Karla says that, ideally, individuals should be engaged in the community not just for errands and essential tasks but for leisure activities, volunteer events, employment, and social activities. She says individuals should be encouraged to the extent possible to participate. Dr. Joette James says the issue is making sure *inclusion* considers students of color.

Public Law 106-402 item 16 says that the goals of the Nation (USA) is to provide individuals with developmental disabilities with the information, skills, opportunities, and support to:

A. Make informed choices and decisions about their lives;

B. Live in homes and communities in which such individuals can exercise their full rights and responsibilities as citizens;

C. Pursue meaningful and productive lives;

D. Contribute to their families, communities, and States, and the Nation;

E. Have interdependent friendships and relationships with other persons;

F. Live free of abuse, neglect, financial and sexual exploitation, and violations of their legal and human rights

G. Achieve full integration and inclusion in society, in an individualized manner consistent with the unique strengths, resources, priorities, concerns, abilities, and capabilities of each individual.

> "Bottom line, we want FULL INCLUSION for individuals with disabilities" Karla Nabors

Include Special Education in Programs

A primary purpose of Public Law 106-402 was to improve service systems for individuals with developmental disabilities. It also outlines guidelines for "Minority Participation" in programs for individuals with developmental disabilities. State Plan Section 124 cites: "The plan shall provide assurances that the State has taken affirmative steps to assure that participation in programs funded under this subtitle is geographically representative of the State, and reflects the diversity of the State with respect to race and ethnicity" (Public Law 106-402, 2000). You might survey your state's disability education programs to assess its representation of racial and ethnic diversity.

Collective Impact (CI) or Community Schools can be bridges to connecting communities with education programs and resources. Maryland MD Code of Education, § 5-223 defines community schools as:

> *A public school that identifies a set of strategic partnerships between the school and other community resources that promote student achievement, positive learning outcomes, and the well-being of students by providing wraparound services.*

According to the Institute for Educational Leadership, 45% of public schools reported using a community school or wraparound services model. Collective Impact, "a network of community members, organizations, and institutions who advance equity by learning together, aligning, and integrating their actions to achieve population and systems level change" (collectiveimpactforum.org) are effective in generating higher attendance and engagement outcomes. However, the model lacks adequate disability data and the application of appropriate interventions. Of the 15 factors measured for a community school (e.g., mental health, nutrition, childcare), none are related to special education, disability support, or staff/teacher services. Without the emphasis on BSSN, professional development, and teacher quality, the wraparound model is not inclusive and limited in its potential.

Promise Zones are high-poverty communities where the federal government partners with local leaders to increase economic activity, improve educational opportunities, leverage private investment, reduce violent crime, enhance public health, and addresses other priorities identified by the community. Educational Equity plans are included in a Promise Zone charter. Including special education equity practices into the charter would designate resources to address disproportionality.

Promise Neighborhoods and Zones award funds to designated communities. Promise Neighborhoods, established under the legislative authority of the Fund for the Improvement of Education Program (FIE), provides funding to support eligible entities, including nonprofit organizations, which may include faith-based nonprofit organizations, institutions of higher education, and Indian tribes.

Given the 2023 repeal of Affirmative Action within higher education admissions, ever so more is it important to strategically target and include BSSN into programming decisions, like those for college readiness or skills and trades. Concretely recognizing that exclusionary practices for Black students is not the intent of the ruling, the USC Race and Equity Center says to leverage the language in the SCOTUS (Supreme Court of the United States) opinion and forthcoming legal toolkits to help resist overreach and misinterpretation.

READING-Prioritize On-Grade-Level Reading

Graduating high school on a fourth-grade reading level is unacceptable. The development of reading skills obviously serves as the gateway to the world of printed information, as reading serves as the major foundational skill for all school-based learning (Lyon,1998a). In his article, "Why Reading is Not a Natural Process," Dr. Reid Lyon, emphasized that, "Learning to read is critical to a child's overall well-being. If a youngster does not learn to read in our literacy-driven society, hope for a fulfilling, productive life diminishes. In short, difficulties learning to read are not only an educational problem, they constitute a serious public health concern" (ASCD, 1998).

Fluent readers have solid phonemic awareness, strong vocabularies, automaticity, an understanding of alphabetic principles, are linguistically agile/have linguistic ability, can apply and recognize grammar and syntax principles, use context to gain comprehension and decoding skills to decipher unfamiliar words in a text. Appropriately introducing text for young children stimulates early literacy. The lack of literacy instruction and attainment limits the cognitive flexibility and agility needed for future workplace managerial and leadership positions.

Explicit, systematic, and evidence-based reading instruction, its orthography, and knowing when they are to be used should be a priority for BSSNs. While "balanced literacy" (where sight word reading and phonetics are taught) is commonly accepted, reading expert, Dr. Walter Dunson, says it is not founded on research. In 2000, a government-formed National Reading Panel released the findings of its exhaustive examination of the research of historical approaches to reading. The National Reading Panel declared that "phonics instruction was crucial to teaching young readers…" (PBS.org, 2023). Orton Gillingham (a teaching approach that emerged in the 1920s) is an example of an evidence-based approach to reading instruction.

Research consistently shows that instructional programs or methods for older poor readers have these characteristics (Moates, 2022):

- They systematically, explicitly, and cumulatively teach all essential components of literacy.
- They are intensive enough to produce significant gains in a student's relative standing.
- They stimulate language abilities through the direct study of phonology, morphology, orthography, syntax, and text structure.
- They respect students' social, intellectual, and emotional needs.

Reading is a Code

Maryann Wolfe says, "Reading or written language (as we know it today) is a cultural invention that necessitated totally new connections among structures in the human brain underlying language, perception, cognition, and, over time, our emotions." Demystifying the science of reading is absolutely necessary. Dr. Dunson says that the English language is a code. Webster's Dictionary defines encryption as "the process of converting messages in ordinary language, or other information into a secret coded form that cannot be interpreted without knowing the secret method for interpretation, called the key." Hanes has actually developed a language training system on this code. He says writing is a "clever encryption system"; students' brains have to be able to "translate and transfer" the symbols and sounds. He says, "They have to be able to pull from a full basket and quickly and accurately use the symbols to make words."

Evidence-based language instruction is where reading language is spoken, and the code is deciphered. Reading is not an indicator of intelligence. If BSSNs are taught the code, they can read.

A Basis for Reading-Based Difficulties and Disabilities
Phonics

Phonics does not cover it all. English is 85% phonetics and 15% a composite of alternative languages and rules. Diana McGee says English is not crazy. One has to make logical choices to cover the remaining 15%. So let us say we get to a large portion of the 85% (which we do not in K-12); how do we address the 15%? How are BSSNs taught to make those logical language choices, for example, when to spell the sound "shee" as, "ci", "si," or "ti"? According to EdTrust, teachers in only thirty states are using the science of reading. If teacher preparation programs are not teaching the scientific procedure of reading, then how would BSSNs (without IEPs for reading, impact areas, and OG as their evidence-based intervention, for example), learn the techniques?

Reading in the Home

- Remind students they are more than their academics–school is a very small slice of their life and family history. History recorded struggling readers like Albert Einstein, Rodan, and Da Vinci as highly intelligent.

- Break the code and its relationship with spoken language. Some students are good at reading but may need help to converse about certain topics. Some students cannot read or spell their names but could whip you in chess—their intelligence has nothing to do with reading ability.

- Remove high expectations and societal limitations and replace with high expectations to allow BSSNs to explore their different learning and communication styles.

Adult Modeling

Fundamentally, the engagement with books by an adult model is inconsistent, ineffective, or absent altogether. Given the impact of systemic racism and indigenous oppression on socioeconomic growth restrictions, the large majority of BSSN parents do not have the luxury of free time outside of work and family responsibilities to carve out time for reading or hold the awareness of how necessary it is to make reading a priority. The infusion of mobile devices with competing attractions does not help.

For those BSSN parents who do make time for reading, they may not have been taught how to read according to the science of reading using "the code" to decipher the Greek, Latin, and many other foundations.

Oral Language

BSSN parents might say, "he has a strong vocabulary," or engage with teachers who overlook a reading difficulty with an observation such as, "he's so talkative." Both characterize the result of a language-rich home environment rather than support reading grade level or justify the lack of referral to Child Find. Speech is a naturally developing process and should be considered in assessing reading disability. In his book, *School Success for Kids with Dyslexia and Other Reading Difficulties*, Dr. Dunson describes the oral tradition of language. He writes, "Historically, the oral tradition was the foundation of the informal education process and continues to remain so" (Dunson, 2013).

The printed text involves concept imagery and word identification, neither of which are inherent in speech. Much of the informal education that we receive is accomplished without the use of printed material. Formal education in school requires the ability to read printed material; "printed language is a code for the spoken language" (Dunson, 2013). In most cases, reading instruction must be an intentional and integral part of early childhood education in the home or a structured learning environment. Moreover, multiple indicators are required to determine reading efficacy. Effective early reading skill building involves the use of all senses, tactile (touch), visual (sight) and auditory (sound), the assessment of how well evidence-based phonemic building strategies and phonics for fluency are working for early readers, and the fidel application of early intervention when applicable.

> Black students who have deficits in phoneme awareness, skills development, and prediction difficulties in learning to read and overall reading acquisition, are cause for concern and would benefit from the application of RRIIPP – Marcy Jackson

Comprehension

Comprehension is the purpose of reading acquisition. Parents and teachers I work with often say, *"he just doesn't seem to understand what he reads,"* although I know he can read the words. Constructing and understanding paragraphs and essays is the English Language Arts (ELA) expectation for older students. However, reading the paragraph becomes a daunting task because of a need for more awareness of or application of an appropriate strategy.

The paragraph's pieces, if you will, its words as a map, can be deciphered. The process of intentionally sorting the topic sentence from the supporting sentences with details, and identifying the conclusion, is what Dr. Dunson describes as a pre-reading map. Parents and teachers can show students how to follow the pre-reading map or provide related vocabulary prior to reading to aid in comprehension.

Try it. Did it help? Did you know that such a simple gem could yield a big difference?

Strategy awareness exists in the WSSN communities more often than in BSSN communities. The more literate the adult, the likelihood the appropriate strategy will be known and used. Rather than assume Johnny has a reading disability, apply the trial and collection of data regarding evidence-based strategies, called an *intervention*. The student's ability to improve in their performance is called a *response to intervention*, or RTI. Parents and teachers: Before assuming disability, ask yourself this question: What is Johnny's response to intervention from this date to this date at these intervals?

Dyslexia

Dyslexia was once considered word blindness. In the late 80s schools emerged specifically for students with language-based learning disorders. International Dyslexia Association, Learning Disabilities Association, and IDEA have all been instrumental in supporting students to receive services and resources for reading. BSSNs work hard to overcome many obstacles to have access to education. Daily experience with issues related to adolescence, bias, disability and academic success can be quite overwhelming.

Reading involves three pillars: Lexical memory, phonological awareness, and verbal short-term memory (I can hear Dr. Dunson's voice ringing that explanation in my ear). So when one or more of those areas is not operating, we get developmental reading disorders like Dyslexia.

- Phonological awareness—Can your BSSN identify sounds to read a word accurately?

- Verbal short-term memory—Can your BSSN hold sounds in his head to read a word accurately?

- Lexical memory—Can your BSSN recognize the pronunciation and meaning of the words she reads?

Personalized Learning

BSSNs have a right to be taught in the manner in which they learn the best. The model of personalized learning has been and continues to be the rationale for the homeschool model, and its growing popularity since the pandemic revealed the capability for parents to be educational leaders. BSSN parents can and have demonstrated the acumen to know what type of learning model works best for their child.

For BSSN students with learning disabilities, including reading and language-based differences, a one-on-one model can be highly effective. The Fusion School, with sites nationally, provides individualized instruction in diploma-track courses for students with and without disabilities. The Kildonan School, a private school in Connecticut, applies evidence-based reading interventions in an individualized setting.

Individual language training is typically done in tutoring or academic therapy. However, individualized or small-group evidence-based reading instruction can become part of a student's IEP. Unfortunately, tuition expenses for individualized academic instruction or therapeutic interventions are generally out of reach for many BSSN families.

R-REMEDIATION-Prioritize Remediation for BSSNs

Remediation programs should be highly funded and applied toward addressing below-grade level performance, learning loss, and lack of gifted education in reading. A parent-led remediation is also an option, with free library resources, school-based tutoring, and other community resources. Reasonably priced services are also available for some parents' budgets. For example, Lindamood Bell has centers throughout the community and partners with schools. Private schools offer extension services. The Siena School is an example; they partner with community programs to extend tutoring to students not enrolled within their school. Helpful also are the parent-led/home-based remediation tools such as the *Remediation Center* by Cardinal Reading Strategies, a digital self-paced Orton Gillingham-based model which can reinforce gaps from pandemic learning loss.

According to the Ed.Gov (Institute for Education Sciences), 64% of public schools reported that the pandemic played a major role in students being behind grade level at the start of the school year. More than half of public schools utilized high-dosage tutoring to support pandemic-related learning recovery. Of the 15 factors related to learning loss, none address special education, disability supports, or gifted education. Determining and completing compensatory education services for BSSNs with IEPs is a necessary recompense.

R-RESET: Prioritize Resetting for BSSNs

There ought to be support for students with moderate to severe emotional disabilities to engage in a social-emotional reset. A social-emotional reset happens when the adults allow everything to stop, removing all stimulations for the BSSN. This stop or pause is modeled on the calming corner, and is a dedicated space, such as a classroom, for the BSSN to calm down and use their coping strategies. On a deeper scale, some BSSNs may need a more sustained reset; this can be done at home-based learning or a residential educational facility. With instructional activities, a residential facility might have relationship-building, therapeutic interventions and activities such as rock climbing.

Unfortunately, residential educational facilities for BSSNs with emotional disabilities are not prioritized. Education leaders need to recognize that an emotional disability (for example clinical anxiety) is a main barrier to a child's education. It can look different for each child, so for some children, it may look like outbursts, and for some, it may look like school refusal.

Here is a testimony from a parent of an adopted BSSN who testified to her school district on the importance of prioritizing residential facilities for BSSNs with emotional disabilities. Meet Jenn, BSSN high school parent:

> *Good morning, Chairperson _____, members of the Committee, and Committee staff. I'm Jenn FT—a City resident of over 20 years and mother to two children in our school system. Thank you for the opportunity to testify today. I would like to share what it looks like from the lens of a mother of a city school student with a mental health disability.*
>
> *Let me tell you about my son. My son is a teenager who identifies as Black. He has a genius-level IQ. And he lives in a city where, because his chances of encountering violence are double the national averages for kids his age, he has witnessed stabbings and gun threats. All this while enduring the psychological impacts of the COVID-19 pandemic.*
>
> *Not surprisingly, my son has struggled with anxiety and depression since middle school. The staff of his rigor-infused middle school was trained in top-notch teaching strategies, but they were not trained in trauma and mental health. His school did not have a preventive mental health program supporting their rigorous academics. In this environment, I watched as my son began to cave in on himself. He developed signs of burgeoning anxiety. First, it presented as avoiding specific parts of the school, then specific classes. Then school altogether, either virtually or in-person. Professionals called it full-blown "school refusal."*
>
> *Because his school offered no mental health services, we tried everything we could find in the community—hospitalization, community tutoring,*

and intense community counseling—for five years. All without success. The disconnect was obvious. How can you treat a young man in a hospital environment to feel safe in a school environment? His therapists insisted that he needed school-based support, at least a partnership between school and hospital professionals. But it did not exist. School personnel were not trained, and when I asked for collaborative support, they looked at me like I was speaking an unknown language. I was able to get my son an IEP for emotional disability. But when we were able to get my son through the school door, there was no one in the school trained to receive him. He would hide in the school bathroom or, most often, elope to come home.

The result? My son, who tested in the 90th percentile on PARCC in fourth grade with his genius-level IQ, now, in tenth grade, tests in the 14th percentile. He has an attendance rate of 20%. He is the poster child for those high school dropout statistics. But, I contend that because his schools did not provide adequate in-school mental health services, my son does not face drop out; he faces PUSH out.

Not giving up, I have requested and won a nonpublic, therapeutic residential school (RTC) placement for my son. But here is the new barrier: The city school district offers moms like me a list of approved nonpublic RTCs. There are hundreds in the U.S. But the city school district offers placement at only seven. And none of the seven-match my son's needs.

You've heard my story. My asks are these: (1) Ensure school personnel is robustly trained to recognize mental health issues and intervene early. (2) Empower them to provide both preventive and crisis responses. And, should a student's needs expand beyond the ability of their local school to address, (3) insist that schools provide an ample list of diverse options so my child can be given a placement that will actually help him.

Thank you for listening to me today. I am available for questions.
Jenn FT

R-RESPITE: Prioritize Respite for BSSN Parents

Respite is "a pause or rest from something difficult or unpleasant" (Cambridge Dictionary). There is no argument that parenting a special needs child can be arduous, particularly amidst the many barriers parents of BSSNs face. Hurdles include bias, microaggressions, and lack of resources such as funding, information, time, and energy for careful recognition of child/homeplace needs and self-care. Organizations like the ARC offer respite services in the form of free childcare for a few hours (or a few days in extreme cases) for parents of children with special needs.

Black mothers are more likely to be in the paid workforce than White or Latina mothers (Kirk, Okazawa-Rey, 2010). Black mothers often work long laborious hours void of vacation and lacking leisure. Making the time and having the energy to sustain nurturing homes for BSSN is an enormous feat, one that Black mothers, who see it as invaluable, find the strength and persistence to accomplish. As we begin to acknowledge Black mothers as that "glue" for their household, too they can be reinforced with more strategic resources such as respite care.

The Journal of the Motherhood Initiative (Beatson, 2015) highlighted that "bell hooks' theory of the homeplace as a site of resistance can be applied to the experiences of the diasporic family." Bell hooks writes:

> *In our young minds, houses belonged to women and were their special domain, not as property but as places where all that truly mattered in life took place—the warmth and comfort of shelter, the feeding of our bodies, the nurturing of our souls. There we learned dignity and integrity of being; there, we learned to have faith. The folks who made this life possible, were our primary guides and teachers, were black women. (bell hooks, p. 266)*

Over time the home, whether a tent, hut, or made of brick, has always been the source of that nurture and fortification, where the presence of Black women is priceless. However, many women need flexible work schedules to look after children or aging parents (Kirk, Okazawa-Rey, 2010), and family-sustaining wages to afford quality childcare and regular respite experiences. Here is a Black mother's perspective on respite, a short period of rest or relief from caring for a child with special needs.

Respite Reflection by JC, Gifted BSSN Parent:

Time is such a precious yet limited commodity. Parenting alone is more than a full-time job. Most parents would agree that they often work well past their physical, mental, and emotional capacity; they continue running on an empty tank. Days are filled with not only tasks that require action, but even when the lights are off, and children are sound asleep, many parents lay in bed navigating the mental gymnastics of planning for the days, weeks, and months ahead. They ponder how to balance children's educational priorities, household responsibilities, and social calendars, and they strategize to identify workable solutions to challenges that children often face in each of those realms.

There seems to be no rest for weary parents. I know exactly what parents are thinking because I often think the same thing. "There is so much to do, and I'm the only person who can do it. And who will take care of my child(ren) while I take a break!" I completely understand the fear and concern that parents feel about what could happen if they are not at the wheel steering the ship every moment of every day. But I also know that respite is critical to a parent's own mental health, physical health, overall well-being, and the ability to continue advocating for the needs of their children. I remind myself of this need regularly. And then, I give myself permission to take a much-needed, guilt-free break. A break may be something as simple as taking a 'school day-break,' no work and no parenting, to do something that is wholly and completely just for me. Or it may be a call to my mother to stay with

> *the children so that I can enjoy a quick weekend staycation at a hotel, or sometimes it's an entire week vacation out of town. When I take the respite care I need, I always return rested and mentally refreshed and ready to achieve new successes and victories for my children.*
> **C. Janeè Caslin**

E-EARLY INTERVENTION-Prioritize Early Intervention for BSSNs

Early Childhood Education

The achievement gap between Blacks and Whites begins as early as infancy (Rippeyoung, 2009) and continues up to graduation (Robinson, 2010). At 24 months of age, Black children were five times less likely to receive early intervention services than White children (Journal of Developmental Pediatrics, 2011). The American Education Research Association found an 8.1 percentage point reduction in special education placement and an 11.4 percentage point increase in high school graduation rates among young people who participated in early childhood education.

Characteristics of early childhood education include quality and consistency. Collaboration among parents, providers, and physicians is essential during these early years to identify special needs.

Parents are encouraged to:

- Balance their discoveries with developmental milestones, family history, and environmental contexts.
- Be assertive and relentless for answers and access whenever they perceive a delay or disability.

It is important to note that BSSN parents, subjected to the same racial coding and discrimination as their child do not typically have the same quality or quantity of resources to win the battles against physicians, specialists, and educators who are restrained by their unrecognized bias instead of ensuring that black and brown-skinned babies' lives be equitably valued for their potential and their right to receive accurate identification and appropriate intervention. Consider the voice of Mrs. Dawn Berkeley, a parent whose voice beautifully articulates the scope of the barriers, demands of the parents, and the accountability of the professionals—amidst the intersections of service dynamics. There are complexities to parenting a child with special needs, such as providing healthcare and monitoring education, while navigating systems of bias and limited resources.

Testimony from a BSSN Parent on the value of Early Intervention

Meet Dawn, Early Childhood BSSN Parent

As a parent, I cannot overemphasize the importance and impact of early diagnosis, intervention and service provision in the lives of children with special needs. Equally important to early diagnosis and intervention strategies is the role of equity in both the healthcare and school systems.

When our son was just around 18 months, we began noticing regressions in speech and other developmental markers. Thankfully, our doctor was able to provide us with a referral for a developmental pediatrician who offered a path and suggested a possible diagnosis I was unable to hear. We were immediately thrust into the world of navigating systems, many of which are characterized by barriers quite difficult to overcome and amplified by the devastation of the COVID-19 global pandemic.

With our diagnosis, we were faced with numerous appointments with neurologists, speech pathologists, developmental pediatricians, geneticists, behavioral specialists, occupational therapists, and feeding specialists, among others. Initially, in most cases, none of our providers looked like us, nor did we possess shared identities. As our understanding of our son's diagnosis developed, it was important to us that we had providers and experiences that reflected our own. I think it goes without saying that the shortage of providers for developmental disabilities abounds, not to mention identifying providers of color or those with the cultural competencies necessary for effective, holistic care of the individual. In addition to navigating an already taxed healthcare system, we were also challenged with our introduction to virtual preschool.

Early on, we discovered that we would not be able to navigate early intervention strategies, nor the educational system, alone. We hoped to develop a team that would advocate for our son, but how might we go about doing so? Faced with limited resources due to the pandemic's effect on my husband's small business, we had to become creative, which, to say the least, was exhausting! We spent endless hours researching, calling, and establishing connections to get our son the help he needed in the form of grants, programs and more, not to mention not wanting to neglect our other children who were also experiencing COVID-19's devastating social-emotional effects. Returning to the idea of cultural competency and shared experience is the simple notion of feeling heard and validated. Thankfully, many of our providers heard our concerns, but often it is because we had to be very explicit about our needs and communicate with them up front and often.

There are many names I could thank and express appreciation to for getting us to where we are now; though our journey is far from over, we would not have gotten through those first years without a solid team in place, one who understood and heard our needs. **Dawn Berkeley, BSSN Parent**

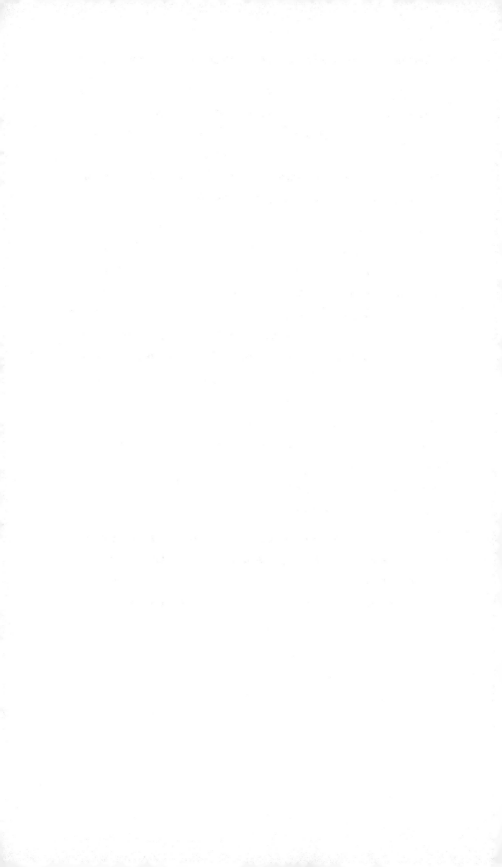

Chapter 8

Universal Design and Accessibility: Inclusive Pedagogical Strategy

GOAL

Given Universal Design for Learning across all settings, the BSSN will demonstrate meaningful progress or grades C or better in all core subjects as demonstrated in three out of four marking periods, by (e.g. March 2026).

CHAPTER INTRODUCTION

General education teachers and other instructional assistants or specialists often provide services for BSSNs. This chapter is a valuable tool for general education providers to learn to recognize the resources and approaches required for inclusive equitable education. Inclusion is the practice of providing services within the general education setting or classroom, also known as mainstreaming. This chapter explores the contexts and strategies for inclusive teaching and technology considerations for BSSNs.

Cognitive Differences and Disabilities

All children have different cognitive profiles and may have limitations or cognitive variations described as cognitive differences. We also need to be mindful of Todd Rose's framework on Learner Variability, where every student has patterns of strengths and weaknesses. According to IDEA law, the presence of variation in strengths and weaknesses such as in verbal comprehension or spatial reasoning, are considered when evaluating a student for an educational disability. Rarely would we find any student with a constant and uniform psycho-cognitive profile; everyone is unique. Finding a way to include BSSNs in general education where applicable is our charge for this chapter. Let's start by defining cognitive disability, intellectual disability, giftedness, and neurodivergent.

Cognitive Disability (aka Learning Disability)

Cognitive disability is evidenced by significantly reduced ability in:

(a) in one or more areas of cognitive function that affect learning, such as communication, reading, writing, or math;
(b) to understand new or complex information and learn new skills;
(c) to cope independently, or
(d) to have memory and attention or visual, language, or numerical thinking (W3).

Cognitive disabilities are often difficult to assess. An educational evaluation including classroom observations, data and records reviews, and specialist assessment is needed to help determine if there is a cognitive disability. Cognition scales can be determined by assessment. Cognitive ability is not intellectual ability (which may or may not be affected) and can have different meanings in different settings.

Intellectual Disability

Intellectual disability is a neurodevelopmental disorder characterized by significantly impaired intellectual and adaptive functioning, with deficits in

a) intellectual functioning, including reasoning, problem solving, planning, abstract thinking, judgment, academic learning, and learning from experience; and

b) adaptive functioning that significantly hampers conforming to developmental and sociocultural standards for the individual's independence and ability to meet their social responsibility.

The onset of these deficits is typically in childhood (NIH, 2015).

Gone are the days of only using one factor (such as IQ) in learning disability decision-making. IQ and academic scores do not have to match. If a BSSN scores a lower IQ on the evaluation instrument, that does not automatically mean a learning disability is present. A psychological evaluation, typically the WISC-V Wechsler Intelligence Scale for Children (now in its fifth edition), is used to assess intellectual ability. "The Full Scale IQ is a score derived from administration of selected subtests from the Wechsler Intelligence Scales designed to provide a measure of an individual's overall level of general cognitive and intellectual functioning" (Lange, 2011). Intellectual disability is usually defined by an IQ (Intellectual Quotient) below 70 and by significant deficits in functional and adaptive skills. The American Psychiatric Association (AAIDD and DSM-5) classifies the severity of intellectual disability according to the levels of support needed to achieve an individual's optimal personal functioning.

Giftedness

While evaluations can provide valuable information, it is critical to not only use evaluations (such as the WISC-V or others) to look for disability, which is a deficit-based thinking approach. We can engage evaluation tools with a strengths-based approach, looking for gifts. Scores that designate giftedness, according to public education academic standards, are an FSIQ (Full Scale Intellectual Quotient) generally above 120 but could scatter across domains. When a BSSN scores high in an area, such as mathematics, yet scores low (say under 105) in reading, it may indicate that the BSSN is twice (or thrice) exceptional and appropriate gifted services should be provided along with supports for the BSSN's disability.

Neurodivergent

Neurodiversity is a novel, nonmedical term that describes a spectrum of cognitive differences, gifts, and disabilities, including learning, intellectual, emotional, and social disabilities, where brains process information differently than what is considered normal or typical. Neurodivergence (the state of being neurodivergent) can be largely or entirely genetic and innate, or it can be largely or entirely produced by brain-altering experience or some combination of the two. Autism and dyslexia are examples of innate forms of neurodivergence. Alterations in brain functioning caused by trauma, long-term meditation practice, or heavy usage of psychedelic drugs are examples of neurodivergence produced through experience. In general, there are more Black students with neurodivergent thinking than we know. Some choose not to disclose because of stigma, for example, or perhaps they are distrustful that appropriate support will be provided.

Labeling

Dr. Joette James says neurodiversity "focuses on a strength-based approach, which only applies to those at the top of the spectrum—not the bottom, emphasizing the feel-good part (of differences and disabilities), not the adversity." This limited perception for our students can be counterproductive as we advocate for them to receive the critical services they need to overcome the negative aspects of their ailments, such as antisocial behaviors stemming from autism or attention deficit hyperactivity disorder (ADHD).

We all have differences in how we think or process and use information. Whether someone needs specialized services and supports to learn or function is where the term special needs are applicable. A neurodivergent BSSN without a disability who prefers to learn from auditory lessons rather than visual presentations of slides, for example, may not need the specialized supports to access the material or services to maintain participation throughout the class duration. Recall Nihcay, a BSSN who has a disability making it difficult or even impossible to benefit from the general education curriculum or program. We would not want to underestimate the scope of his needs.

While the term neurodiverse is perceived as an inclusive description of disability or special needs, it must reflect the depth of support BSSNs may need. A neurodivergent BSSN with dyslexia, like Sarah, will need visual materials in a layout that helps her follow and understand the content without getting overwhelmed. She would benefit from having small, short chunks of content, sections, or boxes and good use of white space so that the visual representation of the information does not get overwhelming. If the learning materials are not designed this way, they will need modification. If creating a modification for students like Sarah is not or "cannot" be a part of the general education process, then Sarah will need accommodations afforded through IDEA.

BSSNs who struggle with maintaining attention or difficulty with memory need to avoid distractions during the learning experience. It will help them to know where a task starts and finishes for them to follow along. It is also helpful to know where the BSSN is in the process to avoid disorientation of where or what the next task might be. BSSNs like Sarah who have short-term and working memory difficulties need learning steps that do not rely on memory; they need to be able to readily access information previously used. This is one reason math computations can be challenging. For example, some BSSNs cannot hold in their heads the multiple steps required for solving a math problem.

Choosing labels or descriptions in programming is an important matter to consider. For our Developmental Driver Education program (Jackson, 2013) I chose the description, "Cognitive and Social Limitations," taken from occupational therapist Miriam Monohan's research. This label best identified the hundreds of students with and without learning disabilities and autism that we assessed or taught how to drive. We found that the students did not always disclose their limitations or disabilities, which affected their ability to learn how to drive.

Ever heard that Johnny hums to a different tune or dances to a different drumbeat? It means that Johnny's uniqueness or specialty is in how he receives information. One might call it a weakness that Johnny needs help to follow the song in the school chorus. On the other hand, if Johnny were taught how to build his own instrument and write down the music he hears in his head, he would be considered brilliant.

Given that all learners have varied cognitive profiles, plan the learning to make content accessible and reflective of the fact that there are diverse learners in the class. Recall that BSSNs are inherently quite diverse and talented, as evidenced by their multifaceted ethnicity, history, culture, faith, and societal contexts explored in earlier chapters, coupled with a unique gift, cognitive profile, or disability.

While labeling can yield needed resources, it can also be limiting. School Diversity Administrator and Pursue Excellent CEO, Dr. Gregory Bell refused to be limited. In spite of his childhood eyesight disability at the age of eight, Dr. Bell successfully completed his PhD at the age of twenty-seven from Ohio State University, and has many other accomplishments. Instead of the outdated 1950s label of handicap, Dr. Bell uses *'handi capable'*. He says, "I am capable of doing anything when handed an opportunity to be invited to have access", an emphasis his parents placed in his mind after his diagnosis of juvenile macular degeneration, which ultimately led to center eyesight blindness. Dr. Bell, renowned for his acronyms and mnemonics, serves as a mentor for aspiring underserved youth, encouraging them to aim for excellence. He is an example to all students, and for those students with termed *disabilities*, he emphasizes that no one can *"diss my ability"*.

Universal Design for Learning (UDL)

Universal Design for Learning (UDL) is a framework to improve and optimize teaching and learning for all people based on scientific insights into how humans learn (CAST, 2023). UDL is intended to denote that the curriculum is at the origination stage, still available for application to all learners. Essentially, it is a framework that facilitates teachers in anticipating and planning for the diversity in learners, such as the diversity we have explored across BSSNs. UDL benefits neurodivergent learners who may or may not have disabilities. UDL (and metacognition) have emerged beyond the limitations of learning styles. The tactile or hands-on learner, auditory or listening learner, and visual or illustrative learners all still exist. UDL is asking educators to not to design instruction toward one learning style or the other, but to be inclusive of all styles.

Universal means all. According to the Center for Universal Design, universal design is the design of products and environments to be usable by all people, to the greatest extent possible, without the need for adaptation or specialized design. Recall how Dr. James described the limitations of participating in norming testing is limited because the equipment might not accommodate people with afros. The scanner is not an example of a universal design.

Alternatively, the curb ramp concept connecting streets and sidewalks, initiated at "curb cuts" in the early '70s at UC Berkeley is an example of universal design. While the curb cut began as an accommodation for people with disabilities, it benefits others in society as well: parents with baby strollers, young children on bicycles, seniors with shopping carts, EMTs transporting patients. The "curb cut effect" identified Dr. Angela Glover Blackwell, lawyer, activist and policy expert, is "a framework for understanding the community-wide benefits of any innovation specifically designed to achieve equity for an underserved group" (Collins, 2021).

> *When the nation targets support where it is needed most—when we create the circumstances that allow those who have been left behind to participate and contribute fully—everyone wins. (Angela Glover Blackwell, 2017)*

In Universal Design for Learning, variability, and diversity are the norm. Bear in mind that all students are unique. When designing with the UDL approach, identify the barriers (aka pain points) for BSSNs and work to remove or reduce these barriers. CAST (formerly the Center for Applied Special Technology) the group that created the UDL framework, does an excellent job explaining the expectations of universal design and what to look for when designing and teaching according to UDL. See CAST.org for further resources.

The three domains of strategic purpose for learning are:

- Why - Engagement
- What - Representation
- How - Meaning

Notice that the domain's purpose is on the learner (learner-centered), not the content or teacher (teacher-centered).

The UDL Guidelines focus on increasing access and reducing barriers to learners. UDL is where culturally responsive teaching finds focus on the pedagogical application of cultural diversity, among BSSNs in our case. While UDL is for learners of varying degrees on the cognitive strengths and interests spectrum, it will also benefit BSSN of gifted-ability, disability, typical ability, or those whose abilities is not yet determined. As you read through the domain descriptions below, consider how you might apply them within the classroom with Black students with special needs.

Provide Multiple Means of Engagement

Learners differ markedly in how they can be engaged or motivated to learn. Some learners might like to work alone, while others prefer to work with their peers. In reality, there is not one means of engagement that will be optimal for all learners in all contexts; providing multiple options for engagement is essential (CAST.org). CAST provides guidelines for Engagement's core elements: Recruiting Interest (individual choice and safe spaces), Sustaining Effort and Persistence (goals, resources, and collaboration), and Self-Regulation (motivation, coping and reflection) that can optimize achievement for BSSNs.

Data that teachers gain from key resources such as student dialogues can be used to design "options for language that honor what students want to talk about and how they want to talk about it" and "bridge the gap that exists for so many students between what is valued at home and what is valued at school" (Degner, 2017). BSSNs, for example, those with attention limitations (e.g., ADHD), benefit from stimulation of their interests and motivation for learning and the ability to use self-regulation and persistence to sustain the learning.

CAST Strategies for Engagement Include:

- Allow learners to participate in the design of classroom activities and academic tasks.
- Involve learners, where and whenever possible, in setting their own personal academic and behavioral goals.
- Provide tasks that allow for active participation, exploration and experimentation.
- Invite personal response, evaluation and self-reflection to content and activities.
- Vary the level of sensory stimulation.
- Vary the social demands required for learning or performance, the perceived level of support and protection and the requirements for public display and evaluation.
- Use prompts or scaffolds for visualizing the desired outcome.
- Provide alternatives in the permissible tools and scaffolds.
- Vary the degrees of freedom for acceptable performance.

- Construct communities of learners engaged in common interests or activities.

- Provide feedback that is substantive and informative rather than comparative or competitive.

- Provide feedback that encourages perseverance, focuses on the development of efficacy and self-awareness, and encourages the use of specific supports.

- Provide coaches, mentors, or agents that model the process of setting personally appropriate goals that take into account both strengths and weaknesses.

- Use real-life situations or simulations to demonstrate coping skills.

Provide Multiple Means of Representation

Learners differ in the ways that they perceive and comprehend information that is presented to them, and there is not one means of representation that will be optimal for all learners (CAST.org). CAST provides guidelines for the core elements of representation: Perception (for multiple senses), Language & Symbols (accessible and shared symbols and translations), and Comprehension (meaning through relationships and recall), that can benefit BSSNs across all learning environments. Moreover, UDL considers that the diversity represented in school learning environments need to "find representation in course curriculum" and educators need to ensure that the "cultural variability be supported with flexible and varied instruction." (Degner, 2017) BSSNs, for example those with language-based disabilities (e.g., Dyslexia), need to construct new meaning through experiencing multisensory content and shared communication and language.

CAST Strategies for Representation Include:

- "Chunk" information into smaller elements.

Universal Design and Accessibility: Inclusive Pedagogical Strategy

- Progressively release information (e.g., sequential highlighting).
- Remove unnecessary distractions unless they are essential to the instructional goal.
- Highlight previously learned skills that can be used to solve unfamiliar problems.
- Pre-teach critical prerequisite concepts through demonstration or models.
- Bridge concepts with relevant analogies and metaphors.
- Provide explicit, supported opportunities to generalize learning to new situations (e.g., different types of problems that can be solved with linear equations, using physics principles to build a playground).
- Offer opportunities over time to revisit key ideas and linkages between ideas.

Provide Multiple Means of Action & Expression

Learners differ in how they navigate a learning environment and express what they know. There is not one means of action and expression that will be optimal for all learners; providing options for action and expression is essential (CAST.org). CAST identifies Action & Expression's core elements as: Physical Action (varied interactions and access to tools/technologies), Expression & Communication (alternative tools for fluency in multiple media), and Executive Functions (goal setting, management, and monitoring progress). All of these elements allow BSSNs to experience learning success.

Information gathering about how multicultural students prefer to express their knowledge is used in curriculum design. For example, some BSSNs prefer competition rather than collaboration to demonstrate skills, based on family and culture contexts. When teachers value "family traditions associated with expression and communication," they in turn "help students set goals that are meaningful and connected to their values" (Dengner, 2017). BSSNs, for example those with intellectual limitations (e.g., Down syndrome), benefit from physical and social interaction with the learning and clear plans to execute tasks.

CAST Strategies for Action & Expression Include:

- Provide alternatives for physically interacting with materials by hand, voice, single switch, joystick, keyboard, or adapted keyboard.
- Select software that works seamlessly with keyboard alternatives and alt keys.
- Build switch and scanning options for increased independent access and keyboard alternatives.
- Use physical manipulatives (e.g., blocks, 3D models, base-ten blocks).
- Use social media and interactive web tools (e.g., discussion forums, chats, web design, annotation tools, storyboards, comic strips, and animation presentations).
- Provide text-to-speech software (voice recognition), human dictation, recording.
- Provide calculators, graphing calculators, geometric sketch pads, or pre-formatted graph paper.
- Provide sentence starters or sentence strips.
- Provide multiple examples of novel solutions to authentic problems.
- Post goals, objectives, and schedules in a prominent place.

Universal Design and Accessibility: Inclusive Pedagogical Strategy

- Embed prompts to "stop and think" before acting, as well as adequate space.
- Provide graphic organizers and templates for data collection and organizing information.
- Use of assessment checklists, scoring rubrics, and multiple examples of annotated student work/performance examples.

The strategies above are best practices to help all learners benefit from the learning experience, including those with differences, gifts, and disabilities. Many of the strategies outlined above can be developed as part of the Individualized Education Plan for students who meet the educational disability qualifications set forth by IDEA. School teams should discuss and identify which and how to implement the UDL Guidelines and Strategies.

Throughout application of these strategies, BSSNs will engage, perceive and make sense of the information to make new experiences that benefit their academic, social, and functional successes.

Along the way, ask these questions:

- How can I make sure that BSSNs are engaging in the learning material?
- How are BSSNs perceiving this lesson?
- Am I using evidence-based practices for BSSNs?
- Are all of my materials accessible for students with limited abilities?

Universal Design for Learning can be embraced as a flexible approach to removing barriers. UDL allows learners to be purposeful, motivated, resourceful, knowledgeable, strategic, and goal-directed. Most of all, BSSNs can contribute and feel empowered.

UDL Example

UDL can be used to help interrupt discipline referral disproportionality. A school district in Indiana laid out a location matrix of all the referrals and suspensions to identify the places from within the schools where the behaviors were happening. Over 95% of the discipline referrals came from the learning environments (e.g., classrooms and other spaces where students learn or receive interventions), not from the hallways, cafeteria, or other noninstructional areas. By recognizing the data at this specificity, resources could be directed toward the pain points. The district considered ways to use UDL facilitators (UDL-trained teachers) to help when teachers were quick to refer a student. Teachers were encouraged not to refer a student for discipline unless they had first worked with a UDL facilitator to remove as many barriers to learning as possible.

Differentiated Instruction

Where UDL is a proactive approach to teaching and learning, Differentiated Instruction (DI) is more reactive. DI targets certain skills or strategies after data is obtained, or responds to a certain learner or group needing specific instruction. DI would afford accommodations for students with and without IEPs. Both UDL and DI are pretty flexible, which is the aspiration. Both will use various tools and resources and support scaffolding as an integral part of the instructional strategy.

Digital Equity, Online Learning, Accessibility, and Assistive Technology

In March 2020, the nation's exposure to the worldwide pandemic of COVID-19 required a national quarantine, closing schools and limiting community activities. After a few weeks, schools transitioned to distance learning to continue learning for the remainder of the school year. Distance learning, also called Distance Education, is where instruction is not provided on-site. Classes may be broadcast or conducted by mail or the internet. A Distance Learning Plan outlines the aspects of the IEP that can be accomplished in the distance education model. In other words, what aids or services from the student's IEP can be delivered virtually, for example? Aids, services or accommodations in online learning that generally can be met are Graphic Organizer, Check for Understanding, and Speech-to-Text. Aids, Services or Accommodations in online learning that generally cannot be met are Preferential Seating, Physical Therapy, and Hand-over-hand.

The Digital Divide

While the COVID-19 pandemic advanced the applications of educational technologies, it also highlighted the gap in educational resources for underserved students. When almost all structured learning occurs online, it is critical for students to acquire information technology skills and broadband access. The Digital Divide is the disparity in access to information technologies and digital services between different groups. "These broadband gaps are particularly pronounced in Black and Hispanic households" (Anderson, 2020). Moreover, inequities in digital services can present as inconsistent or in limited broadband connections. For underserved students with special needs, acquiring information technology skills can be troubling. For a child with an emotional disability, for example, frustrations with broadband can increase anxiety, decreasing the ability to attend to learning.

> *At the onset of the pandemic, only 67% of K–12 students had reliable access to computing devices; access levels were deficient among low-income (52%), Black (58%), and Latino (61%) students. As schools shifted online, the digital divide may have worsened other inequities. Many students—particularly English Learners and those with disabilities—rely on schools for occupational therapy, academic and social support, mental health care, and other services. (Public Policy in California)*

Accessibility

The digital divide is not just in terms of internet access but also in ensuring that the digital content is usable by all. Accessibility "means that people with disabilities can equally perceive, understand, navigate, and interact with online courses, including tools and materials. It also means they can contribute equally without barriers and discriminatory aspects related to equivalent user experience for people with disabilities" (Web Accessibility Initiative-WAI). According to the Assistive Technology Industry Association (ATIA), products, equipment, and systems that enhance learning, working, and daily living for persons with disabilities are defined as Assistive Technology (AT). ATIA says that the variety of AT is broad. For example, AT can be low-tech, such as communication boards made of cardboard or fuzzy felt, and high-tech, such as special-purpose computers or software. Another broad but useful framework is by Quality Matters, Inc., which provides accessibility-specific review standards in the evaluation of the online course design's ability to promote access for learners with disabilities.

BSSNs with cognitive and learning disabilities will need systems of support and practices to be successful in the digital learning environment. UDL promotes the proactive process of designing with accessibility in mind. WAI has provided clear guidance for content designers and AT specialists to test the digital environment with applications and real users to ensure suitability. WAI emphasizes the importance of online learning applications and learning management system design teams to help users (in this case BSSN) within the digital environment to:

- Understand what things are and how to use them,
- Be able to find what they need,
- Experience clear context in terms of text, images, and media,
- Avoid mistakes,

- Focus,
- Ensure that processes do not rely on memory,
- Access help and support,
- Adapt and personalize.

For example, a BSSN with a brain like Nihcay's might "shut down" (because of cognitive overload) after viewing complex images and text, keeping him from following and processing the information presented. Using a good amount of white space and still, simple digital graphics will help Nihcay. A BSSN like Sarah might struggle to keep track of complex tasks. In her case, she will need to have the task steps displayed and the use of digital breadcrumbs, arrows, and completion markers embedded. The technologies and related resources to help BSSNs like Nihcay and Sarah, exist and need to be provided.

Assistive Technology

Assistive technologists can assess the accessibility of a learning platform for learners with impairments such as speech, vision, or hearing. For students with visual impairments, designers can create meaningful hyperlinks so that the screen readers can inform the learner what the purpose of the hyperlink is. So, for example, do not use "visit: http://specialeducationequity.html" because the screen readers will read those letters to the BSSN who has limited or no vision; instead, create a link such as "read about special education equity before you begin your advocacy work." Likewise, providing alternate textual (alt-text) representation of the graphic images in your platform or online course site will allow the limited or no vision BSSN to recognize your description. For example, the alt-text could be described as "a black boy with a red shirt and black helmet sitting on a blue 10-speed bicycle" for an image of a Black boy on a bicycle.

Assistive technologists are expected to be culturally competent when using assistive technologies and Augmentative and Alternative Communication (AAC). Research from the University of Manitoba discovered that the values that current AAC practices embrace are based upon a Western ideology that favors autonomy, independence, and self-determinism (Ripat & Woodgate, 2010). Likewise AT practices can favor cultural bias rather than cultural reciprocity, where "service providers tease out the underpinnings of their own set of beliefs and values rather than assume that they represent a universal belief system." (Ripat & Woodgate, 2011). Embracing "cultural reciprocity" allows the provider to take the family's cultural perspective on disability and the use of AAC and find tools and an intervention plan to meet the linguistic and cultural needs of the user (Ripat & Woodgate, 2011).

Universal Design for Learning, Accessibility, and Assistive Technology are widely researched methodologies for including all students within the learning content. For BSSNs it proves to be an equitable opportunity to benefit from general instruction. For BSSNs who need specialized accommodations in the general education setting or an alternate learning environment altogether, special education is explored in the next chapter through the lens of advocacy.

Reflection Questions

Choose one of the following questions to answer and share your response with at least two colleagues.

How can UDL implementation help address behavior challenges of BSSNs in your school or learning program?

How are your BSSNs impacted by digital inequity, and who can you involve to help make it equitable?

Chapter 9

Special Education Advocacy: Make Advocacy Accessible

GOAL

Given the RRIIPP (Recognize, Refer, Intervene, Identify, Place, and Progress) strategy and evidence-based interventions have been applied with fidelity, BSSNs home, health, and education systems will demonstrate meaningful and measurable progress in five out of ten cases of disability misidentification and special education disproportionality by (e.g. March 2026) as measured by local data comparisons.

CHAPTER INTRODUCTION

Addressing the disparity in access to special education advocacy is another solution to the disproportionality problem. Synchronizing from various definitions, advocacy means "to actively, consistently, and publicly recommend or propose through speaking, writing, or arguing for what is best for a person or cause" (Random House, Merriam-Webster, and Oxford Dictionaries). Black, Indigenous, and Latinx persons need advocacy, given the persistent and systemic oppression experienced over hundreds of years in America, as described in former chapters. Black persons, in particular, continue to face hate crimes (e.g., murders) and a lack of quality healthcare (Chapters 3 and 5). In schools, they receive an inordinate amount of discipline and not enough education intervention (Chapters 3 and 4).

These systemic issues impact school system issues. Lack of proper response to intervention, lack of proper identification, and lack of proper inclusion, inhibit the general education success for BSSNs. Special Education Advocacy holds school teams accountable to FAPE and fidelity. Advocates with cultural competence, trauma-informed practice, and a strong will to make a difference in the lives of BSSN will be needed for this type of special education equity work. Demonstrating professional competencies and practices outlined in this book is highly recommended.

Advocacy

Advocacy is an underutilized and underfunded yet highly effective way to help ensure that RRIIPP process (Recognition, Referral, Intervention, Identification, Placement, and Progression) happens effectively. A professional can perform the advocacy function as an education consultant, educator or teacher, or parent advocate. An advocate argues for a cause, and is a supporter or a defender. Advocates can be volunteer or professional providers. Expert advocates and attorneys help when representation is needed in a consulting capacity to claim appropriate identification and services. The first point of contact should be administrators and staff at schools who can clarify data, recommend interventions, and facilitate educator communications for parents. Enlisting the help of an appropriate expert advocate can help with forming an expert opinion to help develop education plans and services.

One reason BSSN parents do not access advocacy is because they are unfamiliar with the availability of non-school professionals who are trained in accessing IDEA law and experienced in interventions and collaborations with school staff. Pupil Personal Workers and Parent Navigators or Support Specialists are usually the schools' titles associated with non-special education certified professionals who help parents. These staff may find it challenging to exercise impartiality if employed by the school district. Let us explore what parents should expect from these and other roles related to the advocacy function.

Teachers

Teachers are a parent's initial point of contact inside the school when there is a concern about their BSSN. The first productive response to an academic or functional limitation is to make intentional observations. Signs of a struggle for students include poor attendance; frequent lateness; poor handwriting; frequent fidgeting; avoidance of reading; disorganization of materials; and low participation. Teachers should document their observations, gather informal data, and meet with the parents to thoroughly discuss their findings. The teacher and BSSN parent would then plan to implement a few changes and see what difference it makes. This can be formalized into an "intervention" if the teacher is looking to see if the student responds to the implemented changes over a set period and number of attempts. The parents and the teacher should then come back together and review and discuss the response to the interventions. Sometimes all it takes is a little listening, looking, and leveraging reasonable tools for a little change to make a difference.

Education Management Team

However, escalation is called for if the series of responses to interventions do not have the desired effect. The Education Management Team (EMT) or IEP team reviews the record of concern and intervention. This team is a crucial component to the Intervention and Identification part of the RRIIPP process. It includes the teacher, school psychologist, school counselor, parents, students over the age of 14, and special education coordinator. The team meets with the parent to share their determination of educational impact. If there is no evidence (often subjective or arbitrary) that the child needs to be evaluated for an educational disability, then the teacher will continue to leverage general classroom resources. If there is a concern for educational disability, the team will ask the parent's permission to evaluate in order to find evidence of educational disability.

Pupil Personnel Worker"

Parents often need to become more familiar with the Pupil Personnel Workers (PPWs) who can offer parent support or strategies to assist with challenges such as attendance. PPWs can advocate for education success and help parents navigate the murky waters of special education. A PPW is part of the school staff, and there is usually at least one per school or cluster of schools. I have collaborated with PPWs for several clients over the years to help with truancy and IEP meetings in particular. Parent support persons, or Parent Navigators, sometimes termed, receive training and may be part of a community organization or volunteers if PPWs are not provided by the school. To this day, I have fond memories of my eldest son's PPW, which was over 20 years ago. She helped us transition from special education Pre-K to general education kindergarten; she was kind, reaffirming, and readily available.

Nonprofit Parent Education and Resource Centers

Nonprofit parent education and resource centers can provide training and support to parents of BSSNs. One example is the federally funded The Parents' Place of Maryland (PPMD), Maryland's only parent training and family health information center since 1990. The mission of PPMD is to support and train families to be empowered as advocates and partners in improving education and health outcomes for children with disabilities and special healthcare needs with a commitment to diversity and equity. According to PPMD's 2022 Annual Report: With 117K children with disabilities in Maryland, in 2022 PPM served 16,348 parents with training and support.

Professional Advocates

Professional advocates should be trained and certified in special education advocacy or law and have degrees in education, plus some significant special education experience that qualifies them to serve as a professional or expert. Professional advocates (like some education consultants are) and attorneys provide an assertive level of representation for the child to access the rights and privileges associated with IDEA. Professional advocates are encouraged to be collaborative and not confrontational. As a representative team member, the goal is to work together for the needs of the child, not to "win."

In addition to being unaware of where to find help outside of the school staff, parents may also be concerned about the stigma and bias that comes with special education labels. IEP teams can be intimidating and biased against Black parents in particular (Chapter 2). For example, when a team assumes that a father is not part of the child's parental representation, or presumes the child has an intellectual disability without any evidence of capability and potential, staff might use condescending or even patronizing comments and disparaging language in reports. Unfounded words like "aggressive" or "unmotivated" are often used inappropriately to describe interfering behaviors. Stigmatizing experiences are painful, as you can imagine, and cause parents to retreat and not pursue key services for the child. If we can help BSSN's to cope with their disability in childhood or leverage their strengths and gifts versus differences, the chances for success in adult independence is greater.

My grandmother, Martha L. Anderson, cared for adults with disabilities as if they were family. Members like Paul, Scott, and Alice had permanency on the chores and chastisement lists, just like us. Paul was a brown-skinned, savvy Black man in his 40s with a small. He traversed the surrounding neighborhoods (and sometimes surrounding towns), drank alcohol, and broke curfew a lot. Scott was a tall, light-skinned Black man who looked a bit younger than Paul. Looking back, I wonder what Scott's disability may have been, given his limited language, lower functioning social skills, and frequent rocking. I never recall being afraid of Paul or Scott or seeing any behaviors that were threatening. Paul and Scott would come and go as they pleased; and were seen all around Baltimore City. Alice was a White woman, who I remember as quiet and being mostly in the kitchen spaces around mealtime. She was quite capable around the house helping my grandmother.

I share these memories as a reminder that children with disabilities grow up to become adults with disabilities. They can be included in the community; even athletics, such as adult wheelchair basketball team my Dad used to coach. The value of special education advocacy for BSSNs with disabilities is to ensure that they become higher functioning for safe independence into adulthood where, because they are Black, the stakes are so much higher.

I am honored to continue my family's legacy of disability service in the area of disability education. Since 2009 I have advocated for students with special needs, collaborated with parents and school teams, and partnered with attorneys representing students. Successful advocates will know the whole child, understand the institutional barriers that may exist against student success, understand special education laws and school policies, identify educational disability, and know how to assess Response to Intervention. Successful advocates will seek collaboration with all the professionals who have information regarding the student's education and disability or medical team and those who will provide the interventions and accommodations.

Representation

A Special Education Advocate should be trained on federal, state, and local laws, policies, and practices in special education to represent a child in the public or private school setting. The Bureau of Labor Statistics does not have a labor title for a Special Education Advocate; Education Consultant is the broad title describing some of the work a Special Education Advocate performs. Not all Education Consultants are Special Education Advocates and may not identify as experts. Education Consultants work for firms, groups, organizations, or are independent. Education consultants often collaborate with professional advocates or attorneys, providing fee-based (sometimes pro bono/free) services. In other words, parents may pay an education consultant to have the school, which is bound by FAPE, to actually deliver services. The irony is that BSSN parents have to pay to get something they are entitled to for free.

Council of Parents, Advocates, and Attorneys (COPAA) is the leading national member network of over 1,800 attorneys and advocates specifically focusing on the educational rights of students with disabilities. According to COPAA, "Authority for advocates to attend IEP meetings and participate in the IEP process is found in the Individuals with Disabilities Education Act (IDEA), in the federal statutes and regulations. Under 20 USC § 1414(d)(1)(B)(vi), the IEP team may include "individuals who have knowledge or special expertise regarding the child" at the discretion of "the parent or the agency." (emphasis added). Under 34 C.F.R. § 300.613(b)(3) of the IDEA regulations, parents have the "right to have a representative of the parent inspect and review the records" (COPAA.org).

We know that parents have several challenges in obtaining representation for their children. According to the Government Accountability Office (GAO), the challenges that parents face to leverage IDEA's dispute resolution options include a lack of adequate legal representation, the inability of parents to take time off from work, fear of retaliation by school districts against parents (such as denial of services or alerting immigration authorities), language barriers, and inconsistent access to information about students' rights (GAO, 2019).

> **We know that advocacy is an effective solution for the disparity of services for BSSN. -Marcy Jackson**

Lack of parent training and mental health crises make self-representation even more challenging, post-pandemic. While some parents may know what to ask for (e.g., related services such as speech or assistive technology), they typically lack knowledge on how to "ask" for services. Teaching parents their legal rights, and how to access or rights or obtain representation through advocacy from education attorneys or special education consultants is extremely beneficial. Expert advocates know and understand legal requirements, regulations, terminology, application of accommodations, modifications, and more in the various school environment types.

While many parents face challenges in benefiting from IDEA, the challenges facing parents of BSSNs are greater and wider. Therefore, Rich and I convened a steering committee and advisory board to make expert advocacy free and accessible to parents of BSSNs. We created SEE US: Special Education Excellence for Underserved Students. The case study presents advocacy as a solution, showing its impact and potential for replication. SEE US was established on the premises that parents would appreciate and value the experience illustrated. It recognized that not all families have access to this service but that it would improve the quality of life for the student and family. Students would ultimately have greater access to community services, high school and entry into the work force, and that it would reduce the school-to-prison pipeline.

For our SEE US initiative, one of our early steps was to create a series of testimonial videos from parents, advocates, and attorneys who are stakeholders in the experience of BSSNs. Below is a transcription of one such video from an advocate, Revanette Gilmore, a special education advocate for over ten years who helps families across the state of Maryland navigate the special education process. Her testimony on the disparity of expert special education advocacy.

Testimony on Disparity of Special Education Advocacy from an Expert Advocate

> *I noticed that many families did not know about advocacy services until they heard about it from a friend or someone else at the school, told*

him about it, and unfortunately, when they explored the cost, they could not afford it. Advocacy services should be available for all who need them, not only those who know about them and can afford them. We usually get really good results when we get involved and provide advocacy services. I want to tell you a story about a client I just worked with recently. The client had a second grader who was being sent to the principal's office daily for behavioral disruption.

The parent hired me to help. She was concerned that her son's behavior was being misunderstood and the discipline was causing him to dislike school. We met with the school team and found that he was eligible for an IEP that will provide special education and related services due to the impact of his ADHD in the classroom. Services started recently, and I heard from the parent that the child is happy about being in school. She (the mother) is not receiving calls anymore, and he recently had 100% on a spelling test they put on the refrigerator to celebrate. Getting calls like that makes me happy. I want to get more calls like that. The lack of access to advocacy services exacerbates the already-seen education disparities for people of color and low-income families. Please help to close the divide. —R. Gilmore

The P.A.T. Trifecta: Parents, Advocates, and Teachers; Collaboration is Key in Advocacy

Parents

Parents should be included every step of the way and attend meetings, give input, and be aware of the BSSN's challenges and progress. However, sometimes parents can be uncomfortable with the process or language used by the team. Leaving out jargon, checking for understanding, and even including a language interpreter in meetings can help parents be more involved and satisfied with the process. Sometimes a parent will ask a professional advocate to lead during school team meetings.

Advocates

A professional Special Education Advocate can be a part of the collaborative process on behalf of the BSSN. Often invited by the parent, an advocate can help refer, advocate, and participate in obtaining Free and Appropriate Public Education (FAPE) for the BSSN. A professional can help team members to clarify data and observations, make meaning of data, review recommendations, recommend strategies, and collaborate on the development of IEP and 504 plans. Through the SEE US Case Study (see the end of this chapter), BSSN parents described advocates as: "intelligent," "knowledgeable," "experienced," "friendly," "approachable," and "compassionate."

Teachers

All students need effective teaching and advocacy. Systemic racism has made disparity in special education commonplace. Black Students with Special Needs have embedded trauma from the impacts of multigenerational systemic racism and their own limitations. Your cultural competencies, commitment to anti-racist strategies, documentation of response to intervention, open communication with parents, and application of appropriate instruction enhance your teaching and advocacy.

What Does Advocacy in the Classroom Look Like?

- Gathering data
- Looking for strengths and needs
- Understanding the cultural identities of students and families
- Putting aside biased opinions to advocate for a child's needs
- Collaborating with parents and families
- Reviewing records
- Observing

- Taking necessary steps to gather resources to best meet student needs
- Meeting with specialists
- Knowing school and community resources available

The A.C.E. Trio: The Advocate, Consultant, and Expert

Advocates as part of the education team may also be called consultants or experts. An advocate is an educational professional who acts on behalf of the parent and represents the child to articulate and promote the unique needs of the student. A consultant is a person who gives expert or professional advice on a subject such as disability education or assessments. An expert is a person with a high degree of skill or experience in or knowledge of a certain subject such as special education or special education law, or a specific disability such as anxiety.

Meet ACE (Advocate, Consultant, and Expert), Rich Weinfeld, Rich has a master's degree in education and has co-authored six books regarding special education, advocacy, and students with disabilities. He is a 49-year veteran of special education, with 30 years in the largest public school system in Maryland, and 19 years in special education advocacy as Director of Weinfeld Education Group, an education consultancy based in Maryland that provides special education advocacy for families of all ethnicities and financial means.

During his public-school career, he served in a variety of roles. For 15 years he worked with students who had severe emotional challenges; six years as a director for a regional program with students with a variety of significant disabilities, and six years coordinating the twice-exceptional program for gifted students with disabilities. I have sincerely enjoyed consulting for, collaborating with, and learning from Rich since 2009. In 2020, we started a new initiative called SEE US: Special Education Excellence for Underserved Students, whose mission was to make expert special education advocacy free for black students with special needs. I interviewed Mr. Weinfeld for *Transformative Solutions for Equity and Justice in Special Education* and have included portions of my interview later in this chapter.

Weinfeld Education Group defines the *Role of the Advocate* as follows:

1. Understand and clarify parents' concerns and goals for their child.
2. Review of records and consultation with all involved professionals.
3. Observe the student in their school setting.
4. Recommend and conduct needed assessments.
5. Collaborate with parents to formulate an action plan.
6. Refer to appropriate related student services.
7. Advocate for students at school meetings.
8. Participate in dispute resolution processes.
9. Testify as an expert witness.
10. Provide training and consultation to schools, school districts, parent groups, and professional organizations.

Power Points of Special Education Advocacy for BSSN

Here are key strategies, powerful practices, or "Power Points," which advocates can use when advocating for BSSNs:

Power Point #1: Know How to Identify an Educational Disability

The type of educational disability, and the severity of its impact, can vary greatly between students. A common factor, however, is that the student is unexpectedly underachieving. The legal definition in IDEA, taken directly from the law, of a child with a disability is a child:

i. With mental retardation, hearing impairments (including deafness), speech or language impairments, visual impairments (including blindness), serious **emotional disturbance** (referred to in this title as 'emotional disturbance'), orthopedic impairments, autism, traumatic brain injury, **other health impairments**, or **specific learning disabilities**; and

ii. Who, by reason thereof, needs special education and related services (20 U.S.C. 1401. Definitions)

Identifying an educational disability involves observations, data collection, meeting with a collaborative team and evaluations. It may take some time before you identify a child's disability. However, if found eligible, the student will receive an IEP, an Individualized Education Plan, which will make the curriculum accessible through various interventions, supports, related services and accommodations.

Sometimes, a student is not determined to be eligible for an IEP. Other Health Impairments are a broad category and could include ADHD or epilepsy as examples.

Identification of Medical Disability. Identifying a medical disability is a process that includes reviewing physician documentation and evaluations, involving observations and meeting with a collaborative team. The student would receive a 504 accommodations plan in the learning environment if found eligible.

Emotional and Intellectual Disabilities. Identifying emotional and intellectual disabilities. This is the most overused category for BSSNs. Black students are 40% more likely to be identified as having educational disabilities than their peers. Additionally, Black students are twice as likely to be identified as having an emotional disability and intellectual disability as their peers. Emotional disabilities are a broad category that can include subcategories such as anxiety, depression, and addiction. By diligently applying RRIIPP, BSSNs can be recognized ("R") accurately, appropriately identified ("I"), for example, with emotional disabilities, and with progress ("P") monitoring, address the associated inward and outward facing behaviors.

Power Point #2: Know the Steps in the IEP Process

- Prereferral, Prescreening, General Education Intervention;
- Referral and Screening Stage/Process;
- Evaluation Planning and Evaluation;
- Eligibility Determination;
- IEP Development;
- IEP is Implemented;
- The child's progress is reported;
- IEP is reviewed ANNUALLY or in a periodic review;
- Reevaluation (testing is considered every three years, unless otherwise needed).

Professionals should understand the whole process, how each stage relates, and when to return to a previous stage to forward the process.

Power Point #3: Value Whole-Child Tenets

Every child is unique and it is important to know the whole child before engaging in advocacy. Essential contributors in the interests of the whole child are the parents or family members and physicians. Demonstrating knowledge of the BSSN is part of the Planning and Preparation domain of teacher responsibility within the Danielson Framework for Teaching rubric. Specifically, it cites demonstrating knowledge of students as: (1) knowledge of students' skills, knowledge, and language proficiency; (2) knowledge of interests and cultural heritage; and (3) knowledge of students' special needs. (www.danielsongroup.org). The key role of the special education advocate is to coalesce all of the information to represent the whole child.

Knowing the whole child means being able to make determinations about a child in an unbiased manner based on strengths and needs identified through an evaluation process. Strategies for getting to know the whole child include: Asking parents and teachers about the BSSN's experiences, observing the BSSN's performance in multiple learning settings; identifying functions of the BSSN's behavior; applying critical consciousness for underlying beliefs and assumptions about the BSSN's abilities, strengths, and needs.

Adapt the whole-child tenets specifically for BSSN as follows:

- Each BSSN enters school **healthy** and learns about and practices a healthy lifestyle.
- Each BSSN learns in an environment that is physically and emotionally **safe** for students and adults.
- Each BSSN is actively **engaged** in learning and is connected to the school and broader community.
- Each BSSN has access to personalized learning and is **supported** by qualified, caring adults.
- Each BSSN is **challenged** academically and prepared for college success or further study, employment, and participation in a global environment.

Power Point #4: Apply a Collaborative Approach Among IEP Teams

The professionals are collectively known as the IEP, 504, and Multidisciplinary Teams. Teachers, parents, staff and the BSSN, as able, are a part of these teams. The team explores BSSN data, reports and observations to make recommendations to provide an appropriate education environment for the BSSN. Collectively, the team, including the parent, makes decisions.

Members of School Staff and Multidisciplinary Team (MDT) include:
- General education teacher(s)
- Special education teacher(s)
- School and/or district administrator (s)
- School and/or rehabilitation counselor
- School psychologist
- Related service providers
- Interpreter where applicable
- School nurse
- Transportation and other specialists
- Parents
- Students (over the age of 14)

> Best practices for collaboration: Avoid taking lack of progress personally, engage in making the best decisions for the BSSN, and share data openly and early.

Power Point #5: Understand Behavior Function

Sometimes you can see what the challenge or challenges may be with a BSSN. It becomes less easy when interfering behaviors in the classroom mask the difficulties and struggles that a BSSN is experiencing. Disruption, silliness, and avoidance tactics are all common coping mechanisms BSSNs may exhibit or feel when overwhelmed by academic demands. A functional behavioral assessment determines why a BSSN with a disability engages in behaviors that impede learning and how the BSSN's behaviors relate to the environment.

Behaviors that might warrant a functional behavioral assessment might include:

- Frequent trips to the bathroom or water fountain
- Rarely finishing classroom assignments
- Frequently talking to peers during instruction
- Turning attention away from learning tasks by being silly or acting like the class clown
- Frequent tantrums or outbursts
- Mouthing objects or paper

Power Point #6: Qualify Giftedness

While we envision all children having gifts and talents, certain characteristics of quantifiable measures of giftedness warrant specialized education. These characteristics for BSSNs might include performance ranks above 90% of their peers, ability to do simple addition and subtraction before age four, reading two to three years beyond grade level by age seven, or having an FSIQ (Full Scale Intellectual Quotient) range of 120 and above. Observing for lack of academic challenge is a shared responsibility of parents and teachers. BSSNs may present with frustration or impatience with the curriculum's pace or simplicity of content.

BSSNs can be referred for Psychological Testing by first or second grade to identify their FSIQ. Sometimes, a gifted student in one performance area might also have a learning disability in another. The label Gifted and Talented-Learning Disabled (GTLD) is used to describe the coexistence. GTLD may be identified under another disability such as OHI, ASD, or SLD.

Here is a part of my interview with advocate, consultant and 2E expert "ACE" Rich Weinfeld:

Marcy: What does it mean to be gifted?

Rich: You would think it would be easy [to define], but it's not. Its students who have superior abilities, academic or arts, or athletic, or some type of other performance. What is superior? That's where it gets hard to define. People define that in different ways. If you look at cognitive testing, which is often used as at least one of the measurements, then you're talking about students who are typical, depending, again, depending on the program's criteria, could be talking about kids at the 90th or 95th percentile, and that's usually minimum. So I think that gives you an idea that it's maybe the top five to 10% of kids in a certain area, but it's not always quantifiable. It's often very subjective. Typically, what we say, and what the national definition that I was part of creating says, is if students are identified [as gifted], and there is variance there, that it's [the variance] [is because of] either the school system's definition or [from] cognitive or academic testing. The old conception of giftedness used to be that "this person is perfect in every way" and now we know that if two people are like everybody else, they have areas of strength and they have areas of challenge.

Marcy: How many students do you come across that are identified as gifted, that are either Black, Indigenous or Latinx?

Rich: There's absolutely no research, and I have no reason to believe that there is not the same percentage of gifted people in every group. If you really look, that's the key point. For the MERIT[1] program, my son was a part of the team that would go into the schools throughout Baltimore to see who was interested in medical careers or careers in science. The students would then apply to the program—a very rigorous application process. Once selected, MERIT would mentor them. 100% of

---

[1] MERIT Health Leadership Academy in Baltimore, Maryland.
MERIT: Medical Education Resources Initiative for Teens, a 501(c)(3) organization.

these kids went on to college, usually the first in their family to do so. In my estimation, they were all gifted kids. Now, what would have happened if MERIT wasn't in Baltimore looking for them? Those kids will not be there, these gifted kids. And when I went to many events there where the kids were being honored, and I could see their parents in the audience, I would just guess none of them were identified as gifted kids, but where did this great genetic material come from? It came from their parents. This is the precise reason why identification is so important, and that is where we get into discrepancies, and unevenness in how we identify.

Marcy: So, do we need more programs like MERIT to increase BSSN identification? do we create programs and bring them (Black students) out?

Rich: Yeas, we do need that, but we need that because the schools are not doing their job; and so I think schools, public schools across the country and every community, regardless of race or poverty, have a responsibility to identify and serve gifted kids, just like they have a responsibility to identify and serve kids with special education needs. Period!

Marcy: So, we have this problem with identification as it relates to these underserved populations having disabilities, and then we have a lack of identification for gifted people. So what happens to these students who are twice-Exceptional (2E) who are not being identified?

Rich: So, yes, first of all, your premise is exactly right; that just like we don't identify these underserved populations, Black kids, these Hispanic kids, we have kids in poverty who don't get identified as often as they should for being gifted. They also then don't get identified as often as they should, as twice-exceptional.

So what's the impact when you don't understand that a student is twice-exceptional? What happens very often is you have a student in your classroom who may be verbally strong, they may be able to answer your questions or tell you all about the topics that they're interested in, but then when you ask them to write a report, they can't put things on paper, and if you don't understand that the kid is twice-exceptional, then you're saying, OK, he's smart, he can talk about anything. Not putting it on paper, he must be lazy. He must be unmotivated. And what happens to a lot of these students is they do become behaviorally challenged. They get extremely frustrated. You know on the one hand, they're smart, and they may be aware of that. On the other hand, they know they can't produce as well as the average student in the classroom. They know they're getting in trouble in school, and gradually they become more and more of a behavior problem and develop significant emotional challenges, and many of their students do end up dropping out of school or end up in special programs for kids with intense emotional challenges.

Marcy: Or, like, part of what I'm uncovering through this book, is the pipeline, right?

Rich: Oh, absolutely! So, what if you were a really bright kid who has been totally unsuccessful in school and you're frustrated there, and yet outside of school, you can get involved in something where you're really using your intelligence and skills and maybe making some money, but now you're in trouble with the law, and you're going to that system. So that happens a great deal in the underserved communities.

Marcy: When you find students who are considered twice-exceptional (2E) with gifts and disabilities, do any of them have emotional disabilities?

Rich: So, there's definitely kids who have significant emotional challenges: Depression, anxiety, bipolar, other mood disorders, schizophrenia and are gifted; that exists. Whenever I see a student with an emotional disability or acting out behaviors or inward-turning behaviors, the first thing I want to find out is, did that come first, or did the frustration with academics come first? And that, to me, happens a lot. And it happens more with Black students, especially Black boys.

Marcy: What did you notice when you worked as the county-wide Coordinator/Director for twice-exceptional students?

Rich: These are students who are gifted and identify with some disability. Montgomery County, Maryland is one of the very few public schools in public school systems in the United States or the world that identifies special programming for twice-exceptional students. Well, as it were, you could not miss the fact that almost all the students were white. So, while Black students with learning disabilities were going into programs that didn't really pay attention to the strength side, the White students were getting identified for this very special, wonderful program the parents are fighting to get into because it emphasizes and develops the strengths.

Marcy: How did you use what you'd learned about the Mark Twain School experience in the 90s to address the disparity in the 2E program you were leading?

Rich: So again, I said to myself as a director, what can I do to make an impact here? I went out myself to all the county-wide programs for kids with learning disabilities and went through kids' records with staff, looking for evidence of gifts in kids who were in learning disabilities programs. We identified the kids who with gifts who had just been overlooked, and we recruited them, if you can say that, into applying for and being placed in the twice-exceptional program. So I can't say we transformed things, but we did make a difference for some students; by the way, Winston Frazier[2] was one of those kids.

Marcy: When you reflect on our decision and your investment to implement SEE US, do you think it could be an example for other groups?

Rich: "I think it's probably a good example of a liberal progressive group that is mostly White, wrestling with what we can do to make an impact on systemic racism. I do think 2020 was a pivotal time for the United States, and maybe worldwide. For us as a group and for me as an individual to really look at: well, yeah, I've always been a good liberal person and professional. I've always tried to do the right thing in terms of race relations. But what have I really done; you know? What more could I do to really make a difference besides just, saying the right things? I think after the death of George Floyd, I, along with a lot of people, felt the imperative to go beyond just being on the right side of things, but to really take some strong action."

Case Study: SEE US Advocacy Equity Initiative

Special Education Excellence for Underserved Students (SEE US)

A Model to Address Inequity for Black Students in Special Education Through Advocacy

Administrator: Weinfeld Education Group
Fiscal Sponsor: International Partners
Founding Coordinator: Marcy Rachamim Jackson

Introduction

Special Education Excellence for Underserved Students (SEE US) was launched in 2020 as a solution to racialized inequity in special education

---

[2] Winston Frazier served as SEE US Advisory Board (past student member).

for Black Students with Special Needs, the most impacted group. Thirty years after the enactment of the ADA (Americans with Disability Act), Black students with disabilities are benefiting less from general education than White children. Unfortunately, for decades there has been a disparity between how Black students and White students are identified and served in special education. Black Students with Special Needs are underidentified for appropriate special education services and overidentified for certain categories, including Intellectual Disabilities and Emotional Disabilities. As our early findings in 2020 revealed, BSSN (Black Students with Special Needs) who do not receive appropriate services in school have poorer outcomes.

Early SEE US findings revealed that:

- Black students are identified as 2.22 times higher with Intellectual Disabilities and 2.08 times higher with Emotional Disturbance than White students in the same 6-21 age range. (USDE, 2019).

- 75.4% of White male students and 45.6% of Black male students receive special education services among fourth graders in the lowest reading decile. (USDE, 2019).

- Due to discipline disparity, Black students with disabilities lose 77 more days of instruction per school year on average than White students with disabilities. (Center for Civil Rights Remedies 2018, Disabling Punishment).

- Black students make up 50% of all students with disabilities in correctional facilities. (Disability Rights & Education Defense Fund 2014, School-to-Prison Pipeline).

- Of students with disabilities, Black students are 1.5 times more likely to drop out of school than White students with disabilities. (National Center for Education Statistics, 2017-2018).

Upon analysis of parent surveys, student outcomes, and data from IDEA (Individuals with Disabilities Education Act) and COPAA (Council of Parents and Advocates Association), we found that expert special education advocacy makes a difference in the quality of special education plans and services. In 2022, SEE US concluded a two-year study of the efficacy of expert special education advocacy solely for Black students with special needs. SEE US formed the process, delivered and evaluated results, and made recommendations.

I. Formation

SEE US Steering Committee of education disability and equity experts helped Rich Weinfeld and Marcy Jackson of Weinfeld Education Group to establish the framework for SEE US. The framework formed the purpose, target population, funding structure, marketing (website and testimonial videos), implementation, and leadership. SEE US formed an advisory board, defined a mission, and validated the barriers to access.

Advisory Board

An advisory board inclusive of disability providers, parents, past students, educators, advocates, and professionals guided SEE US from 2020 to 2022. The Advisory Board developed the SEE US mission, goals, and timeline, and met quarterly in year one and biannually in year two. We carefully sought and engaged a blend of Black and White business leaders, parents, educators, and equity professionals to serve on our advisory board: Attorney Jani Tillery, JD (President); Retired Special Education Director Gwendolyn Mason (Vice President); BSSN Parent and Physician, Joanne Phelps, MD (Secretary); Civil Rights Attorney Gary Gilbert, JD; CEO of Minds Matter, Patrick Corvington; Neuropsychologist, Joette James, PhD; Professor of Black Studies, Norrell Edwards, PhD; CEO of Barbour Group, Karen Barbour; Kingsbury Wellness & Learning Group Executive Director, Elliot Conklin, PsyD; and CEO of Danae and former BSSN Winston Frazer;

Management Executive and BSSN parent, C. Janeè Caslin, MBA; and CEO and Philanthropist, Robin Salomon.

Board members met quarterly/biannually as a group and more often for certain activities. Here is what two board members, Joette James, PhD and Gary Gilbert, JD, shared for why they joined SEE US:

> I joined because I see firsthand the long-term impact of systemic racism on children of color, especially individuals with developmental disabilities. I work in a forensic context, and the school-to-prison pipeline is real. I wanted to be a part of a group that intervenes in a concrete and practical way before it is too late.

Joette James, PhD
Neuropsychologist, SEE US Advisory Board Member

> It is very rewarding to be part of the SEE US mission. The failure to meet the educational needs of children with special needs is a chronic problem in the U.S., and those families who have been impacted by systemic racism face additional barriers in finding expert, special education advocacy. Enabling these families to obtain educational advocacy so that the child can have the opportunities to succeed in school is an especially satisfying experience.

Gary Gilbert

Attorney, SEE US Advisory Board Member

Mission

The SEE US mission provided free Expert Special Education Advocacy to Black students with special needs in the Metropolitan DC region whose parents identified the child as Black and who could recognize how the family's life has been impacted by systemic racism. The SEE

US mission targets the (special education) effects of systemic racism on BSSN who:

- Identify as Black
- Are not receiving appropriate special education services;
- Are victims of or living with families that have suffered historic oppression (such as slavery, hate crimes, and mass incarceration);
- Are at any socioeconomic level (financial need of the student's family was not considered in 2020-2022);
- Reside in the DC, Maryland, and/or Northern Virginia region;
- Attend public, private, or parochial schools Pre-K through 12th grade;
- Were referred by partners, colleagues, past clients, or through social media and websites.

Barriers to Access

SEE US began in 2020 with the recognition that there were five key barriers (identified by the Government Accountability Office) that parents of Black Students with Special Needs faced when accessing advocacy services. The data from this two-year study validated our early research. Parents cited that the following barriers were removed as a result of SEE US: Concerns around stigma about special education (13%), the uncertainty of the process to follow to receive services (37%), and information/knowledge about how to advocate for their child (43%).

The following are reasons parents had not used advocacy prior to SEE US:

- Cost for service (72%)

- Awareness of service (62%)
- Other (43%)
- Uncertainty of the process (37%)
- Stigma (13%)

Following is a sample of intake comments from SEE US specialists that support evidence of barriers to access:

- The first time that mom asked for an IEP in first grade for her child, she did not know anything about advocacy and did not know about the process. So, she did not receive an IEP until third grade after severe difficulty, especially in remote learning, which went from being challenging to overwhelming.
- Mom is a special education teacher and tried to do it on her own. The stigma is that she is a professional and should know already.
- Cost is the main barrier to services. However, the family has done what is necessary to ensure proper services for the child. The school has done psychological and educational assessments, but the parent does not believe that testing represents the true levels of the child. Some services have been discontinued that the parents believe should not have been.
- It took suspension for the school to take her seriously.

II. Delivery & Results

Services Delivered and Evaluated for (A) Intake

Thirty SEE US Clients were serviced through a contracted provider and initial benefactor Weinfeld Education Group. SEE US raised $20,000 from donations through fiscal sponsor International Partners and company matches. SEE US supplied free advocacy to 30 parents: There are eight closed cases and 22 ongoing at the time of this report. Portions of the advocacy service were completed during the emergency remote learning situation because of the global public health pandemic.

SEE US Clients received personalized intakes where they expressed their concerns and frustrations and personal details of how the child has been impacted by systemic racism and overlooked by school services.

SEE US Clients received three-hour advocacy services, beginning with an in-depth exploration of the child's educational history through parent discussion and review of records such as IEP or 504 Plan, evaluations, reports, etc., and conference with parents/teachers. In some cases, classroom observations of the student were performed, depending on the case situation and remaining allowance of the three-hour allocation. In some cases, up to 15 hours of service was granted upon request based on case severity or need for additional services such as triennial IEP reevaluation preparation, manifestation meetings, progress monitoring, legal intervention, assessment referral, and/or extreme financial need.

The following is a list of services that SEE US Clients received:

- Classroom observations (73%)
- Recommendations via parent meetings (87%)
- Record reviews (100%)
- Continuation clauses* (75%)

*SEE US Clients received recommendations for the next steps to be executed by either the parent or the school. They included changes to IEP goals, accommodations, or services; exploration for change of placement; and application of progress monitoring.

A-Intake Data: Onboarding Clients and Initiating Services

SEE US administered personal screenings via telephone and assisted parents in completing the intake process forms for 30 parents to facilitate applying for services, given the impact that trauma from systemic racism has had on executive functioning. Intake data revealed the following:

- 93% Identified as Black (one did not qualify as Black)
- 60% Impacted by systemic racism in the form of healthcare
- 56% Impacted by systemic racism in the form of housing
- 56% Impacted by systemic racism in the form of incarceration
- 50% fifth and ninth grades
- 25% G school district
- 14.8% M school district
- 90% Existing disability*
- 73% IEP (Individual Education Plan)
- 13% 504 plan
- 6.7% No IEP / No education plan
- 53% autism
- 50% ADHD
- 50% other**
- 13% Intellectual disability
- 13% Emotional disability*
- 6.7% Gifted & talented*
- 59.3% Parents believed their child was in danger of harm: 70% cited emotional harm and 30% other, if the child continued in

school without appropriate support. Harm types included expulsion, traumatic experience, failure of the school to follow the written plan, the child not being in school, parental distress because of the school situation, and unfinished learning due to the pandemic.

*Black students with special needs are reportedly disproportionately underidentified as gifted & talented and over-identified as having an emotional disabiity

**Visual impairment, developmental delay, vision, dyslexia, speech impediment, epilepsy, fetal alcohol disorder, and OHI (Other Health Impairment)

Following is a sample of initial parental concerns captured during the intake process:

- "School changed coding without parent permission. Mood regulation disorder and depressive disorder. Adaptive disorder. A parent needs an advocate to work with her in contacting the school and setting up and attending IEP meetings. There are so many changes that have been made without IEP meetings or parents' consent. The parent would like for a student to be in a school capable of meeting all her needs." **BSSN Parent A**

- "No services have been provided for a child this school year. Mom has filed papers with county special education department. School teachers were unaware that the student was identified with autism. The IEP meeting stopped because the school said they had no information on his needs after three quarters of the school year. Numerous difficulties with school. The child was out of school for three weeks because the child's records were mixed up. Needs an advocate to assist with setting up and attending meetings. The child appears to have been "lost" in system records and identifications." **BSSN Parent B**

- "School transfer due to expulsion from the private placement. The student is not allowed back in school; transfer pending; IEP meeting date is 2/14/22." **BSSN Parent C**

- "Immediate educational assessments. Schools are trying to "boot" students." **BSSN Parent D**

B-Outcomes of Delivery: The Experience of Advocacy and Administration during and because of Advocacy Services

SEE US coordinated advocacy services for 28 students. Services were provided to ensure that Black students with special needs were receiving appropriate special education services and interventions. Services included: Helping parents understand recent testing results and how those should impact current and future school plans; working with the current school to improve the accommodations plan; in-person classroom observations; and several meetings to gather data and to develop, review, or revise the IEP or 504 plans.

Overall, a 55% positive change for clients was reported by advocates. Across the clientele, additional supports and goals were added to student IEPs. SEE US explored and provided a number of advocacy and relational services to support the mission. However, there were some activities and services that, while approved, were not implemented. Following are examples of client advocacy outcomes:

- 66% reported that the SEE US experience improved the quality of life for the students.

- 33% reported that their child enjoys going to school for the first time.

- Three students who did not have special education services before SEE US were evaluated and started new special education services.

- One client disability code was changed from OHI to ID
- One client had services changed from inside general education to outside general education.
- School provided tutoring, 1:1 paraeducator, and social skills training.
- Secured updated evaluations, such as Speech & Language, more social-emotional goals and supports, including counseling, and added life skills goals.
- Better communication with staff, updated evaluations, better developed IEP goals, services, accommodations, measurable goals, and life skills accommodations.
- No longer needed advocacy.

Parents had comments at the conclusion of service:

- "Your program was a godsend for us…" **SEE US, Parent 2022**
- "The teachers and administration didn't know what to do with my child. They blew me off a lot because she was in her final year at that school. With the advocate, they were more responsive to my communications and requests for meetings and evaluations." **SEE US, Parent 2022**
- "I simply wanted to thank our advocate and the SEE US program for making available what I knew our family did not have access to at such a critical time." **SEE US, Parent 2021**

Advocates also reflected about parent knowledge, engagement, and concerns upon conclusion of service:

- The parent is more informed about the son's rights and the IEP process. The parent did not want her son to attend a specific high school in X County, so the parent decided to unilaterally place him in a private school.

- I think the positive change happened with the parent as she became more informed and increased her confidence with meetings. However, she did not change or was not open to recommendations that veered from what she wanted from the beginning.

- The parent is a special education teacher, yet her knowledge pertains to a different state, with different regulations, so informing her of state regulations was important. However, she would come and go off the radar and return to her background in special education instead of using our resources.

- The mother became emotionally impacted and withdrew the child from the school system because the school was unwilling to change to a private placement.

- The parent was heavily impacted by mental health, demonstrating consistent patterns of instability and emotional dysregulation. The parent made numerous scheduling/meeting changes and communication breakdowns and demonstrated inappropriate coping methods. Affordability is also an issue for this parent to travel out of state to visit a new residential placement.

- A very knowledgeable and organized parent who was a professional teacher.

- I felt the parents were looking for their advocate to take a particular stance that aligned with their thinking. I cannot definitively say, but I got the impression from the parents that my findings did not align with what they were looking for, and as a result they became busy/unresponsive.

- "At the point we started working together, he (student) was about to enter high school, and his mom had already given up on the system. I continue to see patterns with clients who have reduced fees, which is the lack of information parents have about the IEP or Section 504 Process, such as their child's rights, and they do not know what other options are there for them."
- "Student stayed motivated to do her best under extenuating circumstances."

Following are reflections from advocated about schools' participation, support, and process:

Public Schools

- Student has more accurate services on IEP, but school is still minimizing the overall impact on her progress.
- The Parent and I spoke regularly about her concern that the IEP team does not show her respect and is not listening to her about the significant needs of her daughter.
- X City Public Schools will not concede to poor student performance even with evidence and X state agency agreeing with several of the state complaint items.
- School agreed to an occupational therapy evaluation; school agreed to 504 plan, but the mom did not agree to 504. Mom wanted his IEP to include more than speech (was previously a Developmental Delay).

Private Schools

- The private school asked the student to leave, and the mom had to find a new school for the student at the end of her tenth grade year.

- The client was in a private Catholic school that was not suited to provide learning support.

While Not Approved as Part of the SEE US Model, the Following Were Performed:

- SEE US delivered four presentations and several interviews over two years to the community of parents and professional counselors, psychologists, and physicians.
- SEE US explored and piloted a partnership with nonprofit organizations. Some serve as referral sources, provide parent education, and provide expert advocacy services.
- SEE US provided professional development training and an online course to schools, staff, and teachers.
- SEE US secured Pro-bono attorney services for two clients.
- SEE US provided three free information sessions to the community.

"The review of the disparity between advocacy utilization, discipline in schools, and teacher influence in attaining services for persons of color (was excellent). Testimonials were very impactful to the presentation and resonated with my family's experience with acquiring special education services for my son and how it could change the trajectory of his life." **C. F., Parent, SEE US Presentation**

Examples of Services Approved for Implementation, Yet Not Implemented.

- Parent toolkits of resources to support parent-led continued advocacy of their child's special education cases during and after funded advocacy service had concluded.
- Free and reduced-rate assessments volunteered by certain area professionals and private schools.

While Not Fully Funded, SEE US Provided Support for or Recommended Extension Services Such As:

- Work with a lawyer to sue the school for not providing the necessary interventions for the student to be successful in 10th grade after being enrolled in the school since third grade.

- Check in after the first semester to see if there is enough information to pursue reimbursement and refer to an attorney if warranted.

- Meet regularly with the IEP team to monitor the progress and fidelity of IEP delivery. In the spring meets with the middle school team to determine if they can provide services per IEP.

- Continued monitoring of student's ability to manage social/emotional/behavioral needs in a general education environment.

- Obtain an updated statement from a private therapist, keep data on school refusal and behavioral issues, call another IEP meeting in spring, request the district Office of Special Ed. to attend to discuss.

III. Recommendations

Based on the quantitative and qualitative data collected by SEE US over the two years, over 20 recommendations were presented to the Advisory Board for consideration, prioritization, and action. Below are a few examples:

- Ensure that SEE US advocates continue to receive updated training on cultural competence and trauma-informed practices.

- Ensure that parents receive an agreement that clearly outlines hours of service allotted, scope of deliverables, and available parent education resources. This will help to promote post-service survey participation, process clarity, and ethical data usage, among other transparencies.

- Seek and establish a memorandum of understanding with professionals for assessment services and attorneys for pro bono services, with methods to determine referral rationales.

- Pilot SEE US at a designated school for the target group to receive advocacy and SEE US resources/ sponsor advocacy-focused school communities.

- Continue training, including making recordings of webinars and trainings usable, accessible, and available to communities.

- Special Education Advocacy is a valuable practice to help the education management team to implement FAPE (Free and Appropriate Public Education) as outlined in IDEA. It should be free to BSSN parents.

Chapter 10

Transformed for Good: Conclusion with Recommendations

In conclusion, redefining trust structures, access to quality learning, and fidelity systems will improve the education for Black students with special needs due to gifts, disabilities, or medical conditions that impact education. Failing to provide special services to students who need them prevents pupils who have historically been underserved from gaining access to the programs that will help them succeed academically (Morgan & Farkas, 2018).

If you missed the preceding chapters, here are a few pointers for educational professionals, parents, physicians, practitioners, and policymakers:

- Once upon a time, in America, formal education was born. Afterward, it was allowed to include Black students, and laws for special education. Oppression in America denied quality education to a large part of its population. Many children with disabilities were denied access to education and opportunities to learn. Systemic racism has made disparity in special education commonplace.

- Schools provide several resources to support culturally respectful and safe classroom environments. Knowing the whole child means being able to make determinations about a child in an unbiased manner based on strengths and needs identified through an evaluation process. Best teaching practices support struggling students and benefit the whole class. Teachers and staff often find themselves faced with a difficult dilemma; either address and demolish their race-related biases or allow their discomfort to erect even higher barriers to student success. Recommended professional skills for teachers and staff of BSSNs include Advocacy, Communication, and Cultural Competence.

- Anti-racist instructional strategies embed critical thinking, teach and model empathy, provide opportunities for giftedness, consider subcultures, and build character. Fostering high expectations is a demonstration of opposition to oppression. By not fostering high expectations for underserved and overserved students, prejudice prevails and becomes a platform for low expectations. Teachers and staff have a deep understanding that expectations impact student achievement. Biases associated with racial, ethnic, and disability identity make certain students more vulnerable to low expectations than others.

- Classroom environments are meant to be safe spaces for the mistakes, progress, regression, and self-awareness experienced during the learning process. Establishing a culture for learning includes clear learning processes and expectations. Culture is a fundamental aspect of ideology, systems, and structures. We tend to be acutely aware of our perceptions of others. We can sense confidence through the style of dress. We can hear ethnicity through language accents. We can see racial constructs through skin tone. Multiple research studies demonstrate that a child's race and ethnicity are significantly related to the probability of being inappropriately identified as disabled.

Interventions are practices or programs that produce results and improve student outcomes when implemented. Teachers apply targeted and intensive interventions depending on student needs, usually identified in an IEP. When Response To Intervention (RTI) is applied effectively, it can eliminate cultural bias. Consider the impact that disparities in technology might have on your BSSN. The Digital Divide is the disparity in access to information technologies and digital services between different groups. In the case of underserved students with special needs, acquiring information technology skills is improbable. Despite an increasing direction toward online education, classroom-based education remains the preferred method for K-12 instruction.

- Teachers must comply with school policy, exercise compassion, and make good decisions as they serve students. Educational professionals, parents, physicians, practitioners, and policymakers must continue to have integrity and ethical conduct across all interactions and investigations. While poverty is not the whole picture, Black, Indigenous, and Hispanic children are between six and nine times more likely than White children to live in areas of concentrated poverty.

- Long story short, your cultural competencies, commitment to anti-racist strategies, timely identification and interventions, and application of appropriate instruction enhance your teaching and advocacy.

As we embrace a hopeful ending,

Be ready with a desire to see us: **B**lack **S**tudents with **S**pecial **N**eeds, *and to rip the school-to-prison pipeline.*

Be...

REDI

- R-Racialized
- E-Educational &
- D-Disability
- I-Injustice

With...

DESIRRRRE

- D-Data
- E-Expectations
- S-Self-Determination
- I-Inclusion
- R-Reading
- R-Remediation
- R-Reset
- R-Respite
- E-Early Intervention

For...

BSSN

- B-Black

- S-Student(s) with
- S-Special
- N-Needs

to

SEE US

- S-Synchronize Health & Education Equity
- E-Educational Leadership for Parents & Professionals
- E-Education Equity through Prioritization
- U-Universal Design for Learning
- S-Special Education Advocacy

And…

RRIIPP

- R-Recognition
- R-Referral
- I-Intervention
- I-Identification
- P-Placement
- P-Progression

the school-to prison pipeline.

A Hopeful Ending

What does the future look like for parents like Dawn, Jenn, and JC, and students like Nihcay and Sarah if we do not implement these practices and priorities?

Reflection

Review the SEE US Recommendations in Chapters 5 through 9. Each month for five months, identify one recommendation to create an action plan toward or perform a related task. Your sequence can follow the SEEUS order, or you can choose your own order to follow. At the end of five months, you will have reflected upon the research, best practices, and its application to your BSSN(s) for all the recommendations. In month six, create a summary of your work and share with the Pour the Water community.

Recommendations: Refinement and Research

Refinement Recommendations

As Aristotle wrote in *Physics,* in the quest for truth, the natural process "is to start from the things which are more knowable and obvious to us and proceed toward those which are clearer and more knowable by nature"(citation). To help BSSNs, states and districts can refine their special education eligibility process with a focus on the following recommendations from the Learning Disabilities Association (LDA):

- *Seeking outside expertise to implement training on disability identification that includes considerations for linguistic and cultural differences*

- *Investing in and prioritizing hiring educational professionals with expertise in cultural and linguistic consideration in identification*

- *Completing an audit of their discipline and special education policies and processes to uncover and address bias within the system itself and the actors within the system*

- *Investing in developing relationships with families and creating an open dialogue with parents and families to better understand a student's familial, social, and cultural background and to incorporate parents' observations into the special education evaluation*

Research Recommendations

> *The investigation of the truth is in one way hard, in another easy. An indication of this is found in the fact that no one is able to attain the truth adequately, while, on the other hand, no one fails entirely, but everyone says something true about the nature of all things, and while individually they contribute little or nothing to the truth, by the union of all a considerable amount is amassed. (Aristotle, Metaphysics)*

BSSN parents, too, seek to be empowered with knowledge of the truth. One such truth is that everything has a cause (Newton). Before Newton, Solomon wrote, *"As the bird by wandering, as the swallow by flying, so the curse causeless shall not come."* There is a cause of that special need or disability in every BSSN. The cause could be genetic, conditional, psychosomatic, resulting from injury/trauma, begun in utero, or miraculous yet inexplicable. Whether that cause is worth the search is up to each parent to determine and explore. As each child is unique, remember that a treatment, intervention, therapy, or medication found to work for one may not work for the other.

America has a history of misguided and unethical interventions. "Treatments without a strong evidence base might seem promising, but innocent families are well-advised to exercise a high degree of skepticism and self-inhibition, and to seek guidance from trusted experts" (Shapiro, 2019). Shapiro lists several nonstandard interventions that lack sufficient evidence of effectiveness. Page 273 of his book, *Parent Child Excursions,* encourage parents to pause when recommendations such as "nutritional cures—including supplements and elimination diets—chiropractic or craniosacral manipulation, acupuncture, and hyperbaric oxygen, are marketed as therapy and treatments for autism". Rather than succumb to "futile quests" around cures for the condition, Dr. Shapiro suggests simply to "prepare the child for the road."

How can you "prepare the child for the road"? Identify two practices that you can start, or two policies that you can implement.

Reflection Questions:

- Why not remain hopeful and search for causation and provide the best interventions for BSSNs?
- Why not gather evidence to create new standards of interventions?
- Why not provide for the BSSN individualized special education services while needed?
- Why not provide evidence-based interventions specific to the BSSN's current levels of performance?
- Why not support the practice of root-cause or spiritual interventions for the BSSN?
- Why not expand the emerging brain-generative science of neurogenesis to the BSSN community?
- Why not make available research on the co-occurrence of disabilities such as autism and intellectual disabilities across Black, Indigenous, and Latinx students?

Further Competent Research into Causation

The Arc, an organization founded in the 1950s to serve people with intellectual and developmental, disabilities, supports ongoing research into causation and development of solutions for interrelated causes of intellectual and/or developmental disabilities. The Arc's joint policy statement with the American Association on Intellectual and Developmental Disabilities (AAIIDD) reads:

The nation must value the lives and contributions of individuals with IDD and their families, while also (a) researching the causes of IDD, (2) developing policies to support and enhance individuals' functioning, (c) providing supports, programs, and advanced practices to implement the policies and meet individual needs, and (d) eliminating the roadblocks currently found in values, research, policies, and supports (The Arc, 2022)

By age 16, neuropsychological conditions are common in BSSNs with more than half of the adolescents with ASD (autism spectrum disorder), diagnosed with attention-deficit/hyperactivity disorder or anxiety. It is unclear why this is the case for Black students with special needs. Intellectual disability (ID) status was unchanged for the majority (>80%) of children from ages eight to 16 years.

According to the Arc:

- "Research on causes of IDD should include research in the four broad areas of causation: Psychoeducational, sociocultural, biomedical, and justice causes of disability.
- Research should be integrated among the four areas of causation, when appropriate because causes are often complex and interwoven."

According to the CDC's Community Report on Autism (2023):

- "Although progress has been made in the equitable identification of ASD, concerns remain around the percentage (49.8%) of Black children with ASD and intellectual disability (ID), which is high compared to White or Hispanic children.
- ID is often seen in children with ASD and can indicate a type of substantial impairment.
- More work is needed to understand why this disparity continues to exist. A high percentage of children identified with ASD and ID might suggest a need for improvement in the evaluation and early identification of developmental concerns in children when cognitive impairment is not present."

Conclusion

As engagement, exploration, research, and advocacy continue for BSSNs, my hope is that they are driven by collaboration, compassion, and competence. While the terrain today is filled with obstacles, envision with me a tomorrow filled with ability. I envision correctional educational classrooms dried of overlooked and underserved BSSNs, and college and career classrooms deep in accommodations for BSSNs. I see BSSNs in preK-12 classrooms drenched with appropriate educational resources, and special education processes flowing with voices of courageous Black parents of BSSNs. Take the first step to realize the vision: *Pour the Water*.

Appendix A
Glossary of Acronyms and Related Terms

See Appendix C for Department of Education, Office of Special Education definitions of these disabilities.

BSSN: Black Student with Special Needs- A Black student, aged preschool through 21, who requires specialized support to learn and achieve academic, adaptive/functional or social success in school; may have a diagnosed disability, medical condition, or gift.

Black: Descendants of the form of chattel slavery (a multigenerational bondage of monstrous brutality) in the U.S., and the Great Migration, who suffer today from its traumatic effects, systemic racism, oppression (unjust or cruel exercise of authority or power) and inequities in societal resources, particularly special education. Also known as freedman

Co-occurrence: When the presence of both a developmental or intellectual disability and a psychological disorder, is determined; also called a dual diagnosis or comorbidity.

Disability: A diagnosed condition that limits or restricts function of eyesight, hearing, thinking, speaking, and/or mobility of any or all parts of the body, and requires augmentation of resources, services or environment which provides benefit of access to the user.

Disproportionality: refers to a group's representation in a particular category that exceeds expectations for that group or differs substantially from the representation of others in that category.

Disparity: a lack of equality and similarity, especially in a way that is not fair (Cambridge.org)

Excited Delirium Syndrome: a psychiatric illness characterized by a sudden onset of extreme agitation, confusion, and aggression that can make people irrationally combative and dangerous (Obasogie, 2021). The Academic Emergency Medicine Journal describes it as a "catch-all for deaths occurring in the context of law enforcement restraint, often coinciding with substance use or mental illness, and disproportionately used to explain the deaths of young Black men in police encounters." (Gonin, *et al.*, 2018) Physicians for Human Rights want it stricken from the official vocabulary used in the medical field.

ELL: English Language Learners

Giftedness: A condition that may or may not include a disability, which enables a higher functioning ability and requires augmentation of resources, services or environment which provides benefit of achievement to the user. When considering the whole child, the perspective of *at potential*, rather than *at risk* ought to be viewed.

Indigenous: People living in a land before the arrival of colonists. A term to replace American Indian or Native American.

Intervention an educational practice, strategy, curriculum, or program

Latinx: A gender-neutral term to refer to people of Latino/Latina/Hispanic heritage.

Lunatic or Retarded: A disability slur for epilepsy and like conditions where there is an inability to control the body and where the person is perceived as dumb; this (and stupid or dumb) should never be used to describe a person with a disability.

Mobility: Children and youth experiencing frequent moves into new school districts, such as military-connected children, migratory children, children who are homeless, and children in the foster care system. A letter from the Department of Education to state directors of highly mobile children states: "Ensuring a high-quality education for highly mobile children is a critical responsibility for all of us," wrote Neas and Williams. They continue: "While these children often possess remarkable resilience, they also experience formidable challenges as they cope with frequent educational transitions." https://sites.ed.gov/idea/osers-letter-to-state-special-education-directors-about-highly-mobile-children-20221110/

REDI: Race-based Education Disability Injustice. REDI is an acronym created, by the author, to describe a call to be ready to stop making identification and service decisions based on racialized categorization, and to remove related inequities.

RRIIPP: Recognition, Referral, Intervention, Identification, Placement, and Progress. RRIIPP is an acronym created, by the author, to define the six procedural stages that emphasize equity to address and align disproportionality for BSSNs. RRIIPP includes data, strategies, and roles for accountability. RRIIPP functions as a reminder of the key aspects of IDEA including restrictive environments, progress, and the Child Find process of eligibility and identification.

School/Schooling: Both an institution and a method of education. A process of learning and management of socially approved curriculum and pedagogy, paid professional educators, compulsory attendance of pupils, and school grouping. (Dictionary of Sociology, J. Scott, G. Marshall, 2009)

Self-Regulation: Self-regulation. Self-regulation is a mental state and process in which individuals focus on goal attainment, including control over feelings and thoughts, and being proactive and reflective about self-monitoring (Baumeister & Vohs, 2007; Peterson, 2006; Zimmerman, 2000).

Special Education: Specially designed instruction, at no cost to the parents, to meet the unique needs of a child with a disability, including instruction, related services, adaptive and other supports, to ensure access of the child to the general education curriculum to meet the school district's education standards.

Special Needs: Academic, adaptive, physical, emotional, and/or behavioral specialized services, resources, and/or environment to help the student with or without disability and/or giftedness to function independently.

Student: Person aged three to 21 in a regular learning setting (e.g. home, public, private, parochial, charter school), with an appropriately leveled curriculum that will yield a certificate, diploma, or degree by a certified or accredited body.

Twice-exceptional or 2E: Where a child has both a disability and a gift. Twice-exceptional (2e) children are **gifted** children of above average abilities who also have a disability like ADHD, autism spectrum disorder, anxiety, etc. Because their giftedness can mask their special needs and their special needs can hide their giftedness, they are often labeled as "lazy" and "unmotivated."

Thrice-exceptional or 3E: A child "of a cultural minority group gifted learner with disabling conditions" (Davis & Robinson, in press).

WSSN: White Student with Special Needs. White students preschool through 21 who require specialized support to learn and achieve academic, adaptive/functional or social success in school; may have a diagnosed disability, medical condition, or gift.

Whole Child: taking into account assumptions about the origins of behavior. Considering gifted outcomes and accessing the potential and the risk of the child.

Appendix B
Evidence-Based Interventions

This appendix provides resources to support your further readings and specific work toward Goals in chapters 5 through 9, Priorities in chapter 7 priorities (eg. Reading), and the RRIIPP framework in chapter 4, particularly on I-Intervention.

Guidance for Educational Leaders and Practitioners

Evidence-based interventions are practices or programs that have evidence to show that they are effective at producing results and improving outcomes when implemented. The kind of evidence described in ESSA has generally been produced through formal studies and research. Under ESSA, there are four tiers, or levels, of evidence:

- **Tier 1 – Strong Evidence:** supported by one or more well-designed and well-implemented randomized control experimental studies.
- **Tier 2 – Moderate Evidence:** supported by one or more well-designed and well-implemented quasi-experimental studies.
- **Tier 3 – Promising Evidence:** supported by one or more well-designed and well-implemented correlational studies (with statistical controls for selection bias).
- **Tier 4 – Demonstrates a Rationale**: practices that have a well-defined logic model or theory of action, are supported by research, and have some effort underway by an SEA, LEA, or outside research organization to determine their effectiveness. *(MarylandPublicSchools.org)*

Resources for Guidance on Understanding Evidence-Based Interventions

- Non-regulatory Guidance: Using ESSA to Strengthen Education Investments (PDF)
  This **guidance from the U.S. Department of Education** (ED) seeks to help SEAs, LEAs, schools, educators, partner organizations, and other stakeholders understand the four levels of evidence and recommends a step-by-step process for choosing and implementing interventions that improve outcomes for students.
- Evidence-Based Improvement: A Guide for States to Strengthen Their Frameworks and Supports Aligned to the Evidence Requirements of ESSA⌐ This **guide from WestEd** provides an initial set of tools to help school districts understand and plan for implementing evidence-based improvement strategies.
- Identifying and Implementing Education Practices Supported by Rigorous Evidence: A User Friendly **Guide at The Institute for Education Sciences** By Jon Baron, Coalition for Evidence-Based Policy Identifying and Implementing Educational Practices Supported By Rigorous Evidence: A User Friendly Guide - Purpose and Executive Summary The guide assists educational practitioners in evaluating whether an educational intervention is backed by rigorous evidence of effectiveness, and in implementing evidence-based interventions in their schools or classrooms, and tools to distinguish practices supported by rigorous evidence from those that are not. Guide Sections:
    I. A description of the randomized controlled trials, and why it is a critical factor in establishing "strong" evidence of an intervention's effectiveness
    II. How to evaluate whether an intervention is backed by "strong" evidence of effectiveness
    III. How to evaluate whether an intervention is backed by "possible" evidence of effectiveness; and

Appendix B Evidence-Based Interventions

IV. Important factors to consider when implementing an evidence-based intervention in your schools or classrooms

Clearinghouse Resources for Evidence-Based Interventions:

- **Blueprints for Violence Prevention** (http://www.colorado.edu/cspv/blueprints/index.html) is a national violence prevention initiative to identify programs that are effective in reducing adolescent violent crime, aggression, delinquency, and substance abuse.
- National Institute of Justice - **CrimeSolutions clearinghouse**, Reliable Research. Real Results. | CrimeSolutions, National Institute of Justice (ojp.gov) Federal evidence clearinghouse that helps practitioners and policymakers understand what programs & practices work in criminal and juvenile justice, victims assistance, school safety, and youth mentoring.
- ERIC: **Education Resources Information Center** is an online library of education research and information, sponsored by the IES.
- **Improving Outcomes for Youth With Disabilities in Juvenile Corrections** | OSEP Ideas That Work The toolkit includes evidence- and research-based practices, tools, and resources that educators, families, facilities, and community agencies can use to better support and improve the long-term outcomes for youth with disabilities in juvenile correctional facilities.
- The **Promising Practices Network** (http://www.promisingpractices.net) website highlights programs and practices that credible research indicates are effective in improving outcomes for children, youth, and families.
- Regional Educational Laboratory Program and Regional Educational Laboratory of the West
  Regional Education Laboratories conduct applied research and development, provide technical assistance, develop multimedia educational materials and other products, and

disseminate information in an effort to help others use knowledge from research and practice to improve education.
- **Substance Abuse and Mental Health Services Administration (SAMHSA) Evidence-Based Practices Resource Center**, Evidence-Based Practices Resource Center | SAMHSA The Evidence-Based Practices Resource Center provides communities, clinicians, policy-makers and others with the information and tools to incorporate evidence-based practices into their communities or clinical settings
- **Social Programs That Work** (http://www.excelgov.org/displayContent.asp?Keyword=prppcSocial) offers a series of papers developed by the Coalition for Evidence-Based Policy on social programs that are backed by rigorous evidence of effectiveness.
- **State departments of education** provide tools and resources for evidence-based interventions, for example California's Quality Schooling Framework (CA Dept of Education)
- The **What Works Clearinghouse** (http://ies.ed.gov/ncee/wwc/) established by the U.S. Department of Education's Institute of Education Sciences to provide educators, policymakers, and the public with a central, independent, and trusted source of scientific evidence of what works in education. What Works Clearinghouse ⌐ The What Works Clearinghouse (WWC), an initiative of ED's Institute of Education Sciences (IES), is a helpful resource for locating the evidence on various education interventions. Infographic for Infographic for Using the WWC to Find ESSA Tiers of Evidence (ed.gov).

Appendix C
Disability Definitions from the Individuals with Disabilities Education Act (IDEA) Department of Education, Office of Special Education

300.8 Child with a disability.

(a) General.

(1) **Child with a disability** means a child evaluated in accordance with §§300.304 through 300.311 as having an intellectual disability, a hearing impairment (including deafness), a speech or language impairment, a visual impairment (including blindness), a serious emotional disturbance (referred to in this part as "emotional disturbance"), an orthopedic impairment, autism, traumatic brain injury, an other health impairment, a specific learning disability, deaf-blindness, or multiple disabilities, and who, by reason thereof, needs special education and related services.

(2)

> (i) Subject to paragraph (a)(2)(ii) of this section, if it is determined, through an appropriate evaluation under §§300.304 through 300.311, that a child has one of the disabilities identified in paragraph (a)(1) of this section, but only needs a related service and not special education, the child is not a child with a disability under this part.
>
> (ii) If, consistent with §300.39(a)(2), the related service required by the child is considered special education rather than a related service under State standards, the child would be determined to be a child with a disability under paragraph (a)(1) of this section.

(b) Children aged three through nine experiencing developmental delays. Child with a disability for children aged three through nine (or any subset of that age range, including ages three through five), may, subject to the conditions described in §300.111(b), include a child—

> (1) Who is experiencing developmental delays, as defined by the State and as measured by appropriate diagnostic instruments and procedures, in one or more of the following areas: Physical development, cognitive development, communication development, social or emotional development, or adaptive development; and

> (2) Who, by reason thereof, needs special education and related services.

(c) Definitions of disability terms. The terms used in this definition of a child with a disability are defined as follows:

(1)

> (i) Autism means a developmental disability significantly affecting verbal and nonverbal communication and social interaction, generally evident before age three, that adversely affects a child's educational performance. Other characteristics often associated with autism are engagement in repetitive activities and stereotyped movements, resistance to environmental change or change in daily routines, and unusual responses to sensory experiences.

> (ii) Autism does not apply if a child's educational performance is adversely affected primarily because the child has an emotional disturbance, as defined in paragraph (c)(4) of this section.

> (iii) A child who manifests the characteristics of autism after age three could be identified as having autism if the criteria in paragraph (c)(1)(i) of this section are satisfied.

Appendix C Disability Definitions from the Individuals with Disabilities Education Act (IDEA) Department of Education, Office of Special Education

(2) Deaf-blindness means concomitant hearing and visual impairments, the combination of which causes such severe communication and other developmental and educational needs that they cannot be accommodated in special education programs solely for children with deafness or children with blindness.

(3) Deafness means a hearing impairment that is so severe that the child is impaired in processing linguistic information through hearing, with or without amplification, that adversely affects a child's educational performance.

(4)

    (i) Emotional disturbance means a condition exhibiting one or more of the following characteristics over a long period of time and to a marked degree that adversely affects a child's educational performance:

        (A) An inability to learn that cannot be explained by intellectual, sensory, or health factors.

        (B) An inability to build or maintain satisfactory interpersonal relationships with peers and teachers.

        (C) Inappropriate types of behavior or feelings under normal circumstances.

        (D) A general pervasive mood of unhappiness or depression.

        (E) A tendency to develop physical symptoms or fears associated with personal or school problems.

    (ii) Emotional disturbance includes schizophrenia. The term does not apply to children who are socially maladjusted, unless it is determined that they have an emotional disturbance under paragraph (c)(4)(i) of this section.

(5) Hearing impairment means an impairment in hearing, whether permanent or fluctuating, that adversely affects a child's educational performance but that is not included under the definition of deafness in this section.

(6) Intellectual disability means significantly subaverage general intellectual functioning, existing concurrently with deficits in adaptive behavior and manifested during the developmental period, that adversely affects a child's educational performance. The term "intellectual disability" was formerly termed "mental retardation."

(7) Multiple disabilities means concomitant impairments (such as intellectual disability-blindness or intellectual disability-orthopedic impairment), the combination of which causes such severe educational needs that they cannot be accommodated in special education programs solely for one of the impairments. Multiple disabilities does not include deaf-blindness.

(8) Orthopedic impairment means a severe orthopedic impairment that adversely affects a child's educational performance. The term includes impairments caused by a congenital anomaly, impairments caused by disease (e.g., poliomyelitis, bone tuberculosis), and impairments from other causes (e.g., cerebral palsy, amputations, and fractures or burns that cause contractures).

(9) Other health impairment means having limited strength, vitality, or alertness, including a heightened alertness to environmental stimuli, that results in limited alertness with respect to the educational environment, that—

> (i) Is due to chronic or acute health problems such as asthma, attention deficit disorder or attention deficit hyperactivity disorder, diabetes, epilepsy, a heart condition, hemophilia, lead poisoning, leukemia, nephritis, rheumatic fever, sickle cell anemia, and Tourette syndrome; and

Appendix C Disability Definitions from the Individuals with Disabilities Education Act (IDEA) Department of Education, Office of Special Education

(ii) Adversely affects a child's educational performance.

(10) Specific learning disability—

(i) General. Specific learning disability means a disorder in one or more of the basic psychological processes involved in understanding or in using language, spoken or written, that may manifest itself in the imperfect ability to listen, think, speak, read, write, spell, or to do mathematical calculations, including conditions such as perceptual disabilities, brain injury, minimal brain dysfunction, dyslexia, and developmental aphasia.

(ii) Disorders not included. Specific learning disability does not include learning problems that are primarily the result of visual, hearing, or motor disabilities, of intellectual disability, of emotional disturbance, or of environmental, cultural, or economic disadvantage.

(11) Speech or language impairment means a communication disorder, such as stuttering, impaired articulation, a language impairment, or a voice impairment, that adversely affects a child's educational performance.

(12) Traumatic brain injury means an acquired injury to the brain caused by an external physical force, resulting in total or partial functional disability or psychosocial impairment, or both, that adversely affects a child's educational performance. Traumatic brain injury applies to open or closed head injuries resulting in impairments in one or more areas, such as cognition; language; memory; attention; reasoning; abstract thinking; judgment; problem-solving; sensory, perceptual, and motor abilities; psychosocial behavior; physical functions; information processing; and speech. Traumatic brain injury does not apply to brain injuries that are congenital or degenerative, or to brain injuries induced by birth trauma.

(13) Visual impairment including blindness means an impairment in vision that, even with correction, adversely affects a child's educational performance. The term includes both partial sight and blindness.

Appendix D
2020 Initiative Charter for Special Education Excellence for Underserved Students (SEE US)

Vision: Equitable access to developing and realizing individual excellence.

Mission: Remove the life-long impact of systemic educational racism, for Black students with special needs, whose families have suffered historic oppression (such as slavery, hate crimes, and mass incarceration) through no-cost, expert, special education consultation and advocacy.

Goals and Tasks:

1. Creating a model, evidence-based program that is replicated in at least one other city or region.
    a. Securing a university partner to study the effectiveness of the program.
    b. Serving a cohort of students and evaluating their
    c. progress.
    d. Reporting on progress through research papers and presentations.
    e. Consulting and collaborating with leaders in another city or region to begin their adoption of the SEE US model.
2. Creating programs that remove the obstacles created by systemic racism for individual Black students with special needs. The program includes:

a. Two-hour consultations for eligible Black students with special needs, connecting them with needed resources and providing an action plan of how to access needed accommodations and/or interventions.

b. No-cost advocacy for the families of BSSNs who have significant financial need and that need ongoing expert, advocacy support. (10 hours of no-cost advocacy services provided to financially needs families.)

c. Operationalizing and beginning the SEE US program.

d. Establishing application process, forms, and criteria

e. Fundraising with companies, organizations and individuals, raising $42,500 from companies, organizations and individuals (including matching funds of $10,000 from Weinfeld Education Group)

f. Providing outreach and training to educate families and referral sources about the Program

g. Providing 50 two-hour consults to families of BSSNs.

h. Providing 15 10-hour advocacy service packages to BSSNs living in poverty.

Appendix E
Interview with Advocate Rich Weinfeld 2022

Rich Weinfeld is a 49-year expert in special education, with 30 years experience in the largest public school system in Maryland, and 19 years in special education advocacy as Director of Weinfeld Education Group. During his public school career, he served in a variety of roles: For 15 years he worked with students who had severe emotional challenges, for six years he directed a regional program with students with a variety of significant disabilities, and for another six years he coordinated the twice exceptional program for gifted students with disabilities.

I've had the sincere pleasure of consulting for, collaborating with, and learning from Rich for over 15 years. In 2020, we started a new initiative, called SEE US: Special Education Excellence for Underserved Students, whose mission was to make expert special education advocacy free for black students with special needs. Here is my interview with him regarding the work of integrating special education advocacy and racial equity for Black boys and girls.

Interview Transcript

Marcy: Can you offer a description of your experience in education?

Rich: I'm completing my forty-eighth year this week and start right the forty-ninth year in January (year?). and I spent 30 years in a large public-school system, Montgomery County, Maryland, where I began my career as an elementary school teacher. I then spent 15 years working with kids with severe emotional challenges at two separate facilities where the students were placed as they couldn't remain in their home schools. And then six years as the director of a middle school Learning Center program. Choose a regional program for kids with a variety of significant disability areas and then final six years as coordinator for twice exceptional students or gifted students with disabilities throughout the county. Then, when I left the county, I began doing advocacy for families who have special needs students and, before long, that led to the founding of Weinfeld Education Group.

Marcy: What was the regional model Mark Twain school and why was it so significant?

Rich: When Mark Twain began in the mid 70s, it was largely a White population. It was a model school for kids who are having school challenges with behavior, and emotional challenges, to come to this place with state-of-the-art interventions and cream-of-the-crop staff. Students would spend no more than two years there and then go back to their home schools. But with the advent of the special ed law (IDEA 1975, FAPE public law 94-142), Mark Twain School could no longer say, well, you can stay only two years, and then go back to your home schools. Now, whatever the appropriate placement is, you stay there as long as you need it, and then hopefully you gradually work your way back into the home schools.

Marcy: What was it about Mark Twain or any other school that make it a model school?

Rich: Evidence-based interventions being used and performance data to support. That is, in my mind, number one in making a model. The second half of using those interventions is that those interventions are used with fidelity. Meaning you could have a reading intervention, and you know it works with elementary school students with learning disabilities. You've got to provide it in the way that it was shown to work. For example, five times a week for 40 minutes, whatever is prescribed. And they're very much just like when our doctors give us medicine.

They don't just give us a bottle of antibiotics and say this is proven to work, here, take it. They say take one a day after your meal. Or, you know, whatever the studies have shown is the effectiveness. The other part of a model school is that they recruit, train, and retain outstanding teachers. People want to work for them and are honored to work there.

Marcy: What did your experience at Mark Twain show you about racial inequity in special education?

Rich: During my time there in the early 90's, I noticed a large population of black students with emotional challenges. Racial inequity became very clear to me at Mark Twain. I was in charge of mainstreaming students back to their home schools when they were ready to go back, and then following up with them and their teachers and school staff to make sure they could be successful. I worked with a wonderful assistant there named Thomas Pumphrey. Together we noticed that more and more Black students were coming into Mark Twain, but the kids who were selected for mainstreaming were predominantly White students. So, in that way, Mark Twain was becoming more and more of a school for Black students because the White students moved in and out quickly. The Black students came and they stayed.

Marcy: What did you do to address the disparity you were seeing?

Rich: Mr. Pumphrey and I did some training for staff, looking at the data, looking at what we could do about it, raising consciousness; we made some inroads to help that. So that was really my first big awareness.

Marcy: What was the response from colleagues, staff, teachers, parents and/or administrators to the waves you were making through the staff training, observations, and data analysis that you and Thomas Pumphrey were seeing, sharing, and showing?

Rich: Great question. I think that there's a history of good people who really were trying hard not to act in a way that was biased. One of the ways they thought they could do that well was to be "color blind." They would say, "Well, I don't see Black kids and White kids. I just see kids and I do my best for all kids, and it doesn't matter if it's a Black kid or Hispanic kid, you know, it's a kid and I do my best." And there was a sincere belief, I don't mean at all to belittle it. But, part of that color blindness was blindness. Do you see what's happening right in front of you? Take a look. Take a look. Why is this school now majority Black kids when it didn't start that way? What's shifted, and why is it getting more and more for Black students? What shifted and how can we correct it? You have to address it. So that that's the beginning of it, The administration at Twain was a very dynamic, wonderful administration at that time. The administrators were all for it (addressing the disparities). I think if the teacher were against it, they kept quiet. They didn't think it was prudent to oppose it, and honestly we didn't ask a lot of them. We just said, here is the data, here's what's been happening, and here's how we think we can reverse it.

Marcy: As you did your fact-finding, was there any reason you can suppose or point to as to why Mark Twain became overwhelming populated with Black students with emotional disabilities, and low return rates back to the homeschool?

Rich: As I know you'll present in this book, lots of data that shows that black students, particularly black boys, are over-identified as having emotional disabilities. Mark Twain started out as, not a special Ed school for disabilities, but just as this model school where you can have your kid who's having some problems go, and we're going to turn them around and return them and they're going to be successful. So that was a model that successful and everybody wanted their kid, if they're struggling, to go there. Then, with the advent of the Special Ed Law, it became. "This kid is identified for special Ed. His behavior is impacting his learning and is a detriment to the school." So, what's unsaid is, "my life and everybody's life in the sending school is going to be better without this kid. Let's get rid of him." It became a very different thing, that we can have kids out of our school by sending them to the special school. And I think that's what happens nationwide. You know, there's lots of data that you'll present that shows this, that Black students, especially Black boys, get identified. They get placed in separate classes; they get placed in separate schools. Once they are there, it does not lead to a lot of progress, it just leads to separate but unequal education.

Marcy: Why do you think the model did not work? We find there's this model, this great resources of the evidence-based instruction with great teachers you know, and we have the students who are coming in. They were kind of pushed out from their home school to go here to help their success. Was there success with this model school being able to help? These black boys in particular had emotional disabilities?

Rich: And as I said, I think it was not a lot of success as the years went on and this, you know, as a school. Less success for the Black boys than for the White boys or for the Black kids, then the White kids.

Marcy: I guess there wasn't an effort to have those kids back to the neighborhood school. Were they not applying the same amount of interventions or was the selection committee not selecting them?

Rich: It's a great question. I can't answer that definitively. I can give you my guess is about it. I think that there was unconscious bias among the staff. Not unconscious bias to say, Oh, you know, this kid really seems ready. Just maybe, despite some of these challenging things with this kid is just is so bad that I can't recommend him to go back. And that is what Mr. Pumphrey and I were trying to help shift. And again, I think we had some success, but not major success, and eventually Mark

Twain closed. You know, if you ask anybody off the record why, it's because it was by then almost totally Black. It was embarrassing for the County.

Marcy: Was it segregated?

Rich: Yeah, it did look like it was segregated.

Marcy: How did you use what you learned about disparity and disproportionality in your public-school experience toward your private practice, Weinfeld Education Group?

Rich: I made it part of my personal mission, and later Weinfeld Education Group's mission that we were not going to be just for the affluent parents, but that we were going to have a sliding fee scale so that we could also serve folks that were not affluent. We consciously reached out to different communities to involve them. I made it a priority to hire diverse advocates, and I think we've done a great job with that.

We have a high percentage of families that we serve that are not affluent, in fact many close to or below the poverty level. And we do represent families of every group, including Black families and Latinx families, a variety of different ethnic backgrounds. We have folks coming here from other countries, so I'm very proud of all of that and I think all of that kind of set the stage for 2020 and what we went through as a company and as individuals after the murder of George Floyd.

Appendix F
Professional Development Graduate Course: Identifying and Removing Obstacles for Black Students with Special Needs

Designed by: Marcy Jackson

Modality: Online/Asynchronous

Duration: 45 hours; Six Modules

Credits: Three

Target Participants: Teachers and School Staff at Schools in America with Predominantly Black, Indigenous, and Latinx Students

Target Grade Levels: K-12

Description: Are you ready to make a difference in the lives of underserved Black Students with Special Needs? Change agency begins with awareness, knowledge, and skill. In this self-paced course, teachers and school staff will embrace brave learning practices to recognize personal and professional biases, understand relationships between structures of racism and special education, reframe empathy for ignorance to strategies for equity, and relegate evidence-based and privileged best practices to the most marginalized students with special needs: Black students. Native American and Latinx students with special needs will also be referenced.

Responsible awareness of special education, White fragility, unconscious bias, historic oppression with slavery, and parental disempowerment will be explored through readings, activities, and discussion. Teachers and staff will explore systems and practices (such as the digital divide) that create obstacles and make them impassable for Black students with special needs. Academic regression, high school incompletion, the school-to-prison pipeline, limited early intervention, and unemployment outcomes are almost double the rate for Black students with special needs than White. Teachers and staff will learn how to improve the quality of their role in the identification of Black students with special needs related to academic performance, disability, or giftedness.

Nonteaching educators will apply auditing strategies for cultural competency and anti-racism in their workplace. Participants will see how decisions and data influence disproportionality and its relationship to disparity in the implementation of appropriate services. Teachers and staff will be introduced to the role of the advocate as part of the special education identification and planning process.

Participants will produce one new teacher or staff process to impact identification and referrals for Black Students with Special Needs. Case studies and activities will be included. Participants will collaborate to produce one new Teacher or Staff process to improve high school graduation, narrow the school-to-prison pipeline, and increase employment outcomes among Black students with special needs.

Course Components: Identifying and Removing Obstacles for Black Students with Special Needs consists of interactive presentations, videos, readings, discussion boards, authentic tasks, and a final project. All elements of the course must be completed in order to obtain a letter of completion and/or credits. Objectives are aligned to the Danielson Framework for Teaching.

IRO-BSSN Participant Feedback Highlights

Participants sampled rated that they Strongly Agreed (85%) and Agreed (15%) to the following:

- I found this course to be relevant to my teaching.

Appendix F: Graduate, Professional Development Course: Identifying and Removing Obstacles for Black Students with Special Needs

- I feel confident that I can implement strategies and techniques from this course into my practice.
- I found this course to be appropriately challenging.
- "This is a good course, it changed the way I look at students with disabilities."
- "This course brought back memories. I feel ashamed to have those biases, prejudice, and racism against a whole race. Thank God that I have changed for the better and has helped me to become a better man. I love to teach in New York City; the Bronx is a multicultural, diverse community that has welcomed me with open arms."

IRO-BSSN Applicability

Based on what you learned in this course, what do you find most applicable to your practice? Why?

- I can now better include cultural strategies in my classroom.
- The resources have already been used.
- I learn new insights about how to identify any obstacle that Black children confront in the classroom.
- Acknowledging that learning experiences can be different for people based on their prior knowledge and experiences is a big take-away for me!
- Identifying that there are implicit biases, maybe even within myself, and using this knowledge is going to be beneficial for my students in my classroom.
- Everything.

- Assessing my level of bias and getting a plan in place to improve it.

- I learned some strategies that I could use with Black and Hispanic students.

- Identifying my own biases and how my upbringing shapes me and the lens I view things through.

- This really helped with more strategies and techniques to help support my Black students with special needs. The articles and ideas shared are very useful in filling the gap that I lacked in my educational practice.

- Advocating for students.

- Strategies for learners.

- To provide my BSSNs with voice and choice.

- So much is applicable, really understanding culture and peoples' perspectives and how to incorporate that into the class.

- Classroom environments are meant to be safe spaces for the mistakes, progress, regression, and self-awareness experienced during the learning process.

- Definitely all of the articles and resources on underserved Black students will be helpful to me in my future as an educator. I can share them with colleagues.

- The differentiation strategies to meet the students' needs.

- I found the resources and readings beneficial and easily implementable in my classroom.

- Interacting with other educators and facilitators were the most applicable to my practice because I got the opportunity to discuss and share ideas.

Appendix F: Graduate, Professional Development Course: Identifying and Removing Obstacles for Black Students with Special Needs

- The emphasis on being actively mindful of the diverse experiences and needs that BSSNs have and being careful to differentiate lesson plans for all these students' differences.

- There were strategies, and downloadables that are useful to my teaching practices in the classroom.

- I really liked the Equitable Classroom Practices Observation Checklist and questions about that. I felt like the sixth module offered a lot of practical suggestions that I can easily implement in my classroom.

- Well, I find recognition of the issues discussed to be most important.

- What I find most applicable to my teaching was the ways to be culturally inclusive in the classroom. I felt this course gave a good opportunity to self-reflect on your current practices but also gave suggestions for future practices. It also gave time to work on an actual lesson plan that can be used in your classroom.

- Most were applicable to my practice.

- Believing that all students can be successful if the playing field is level. I did not feel this way before.

- I found the communication with families to be most helpful. It was nice to reflect on the responses of others.

- I believe the entire course focused on anti-bias teaching, and that is so important for all teachers and students. This course helped me to look more at the whole child rather than just behaviors in the classroom. I used our whole child program to find important details about my students and what could be affecting their behaviors.

- I learned that Black students are marginalized at a higher rate than their classroom peers. This information will assist me in making more educated decisions when dealing with students, especially those of diverse ethnic backgrounds.
- Examining explicit bias and cultural competence. These are most applicable as they have given me important strategies on how I can be a better teacher and help black students with special needs as well as all students.

Most common strategies applied, implemented, or attempted to apply or implement after course completion:

- Applied the idea of best teaching and advocate practices to classrooms to better support struggling students reach their potential
- Chose equitable and easy to implement classroom management practices as a strategy for inclusion.
- Explored conscious and unconscious bias in working with racially diverse staff and students

After having attempted and implemented some of the strategies, what is your perception of the barriers?

- "I find it difficult to be part of a system that is broken, and it feels like I am a hamster running on a wheel."
  Related Services Specialist, IRO-BSSN Participant
- "These (barriers) were more self-reflective and discussed collaboratively with my co-teacher to implement necessary changes." **Teacher, IRO-BSSN Participant**

Appendix G
Interview with Professor Dr. Norell Edwards

*(Past Advisor for the Education Policy Committee
for the MD Moore-Miller Administration)*

Teacher Preparation is an essential element in the work of transformation for justice and equity in special education. I had the pleasure of interviewing Dr. Norell Edwards of Le Moyne College. Dr. Norell Edwards is a scholar of Black Literature and Race, a tenure-track Assistant Professor of English, and the 75th Anniversary Endowed Professor of the Humanities at Le Moyne College in Syracuse, New York. Dr. Edwards has called Silver Spring, Maryland her home and most recently served as the Advisor for the Maryland Education Policy Committee for the Moore-Miller Administration. She has served on several boards and worked on several projects related to education. I met Dr. Edwards when she was Assistant Director of Education for Georgetown University Prisons and Justice Initiative.

I asked Dr. Edwards what has changed and what remains the same regarding race and education over the past 20 years. Here was part of her response:

> *We know that the U.S. is becoming more diverse right, becoming more people of color. But our education systems have not caught up to that at all. I had a position for a program on education policy maybe five years or so ago. The curriculum is one of the main things (that hasn't changed). I was always saying, stop assigning Huck-Finn (The Adventures of Huckleberry Finn by Mark Twain). In terms of the diversity that you see in the curriculum and thinking about students being able to really engage with literature and see themselves reflected in materials—it just isn't there. It is so important to think about what*

is shaping student identities right now, how they're maturing; it is critical for them to really see literature that engages them, that gets them to think about their history, about how they are part of the changing sociopolitical dynamics and our world. All of those things are really important.

… And that's also because we don't have enough experts. I've done work with and been a beneficiary of pipeline programs to diversify the professoriate, to get more Black and Brown teachers, right? But even those programs, (you know, we can think about the way the economy is shifted and inflation has increased) the problem is that it's incredibly difficult for students coming out of what we know is a historic racialized wealth gap to become professionals. Because so much of becoming a professional is about certainly putting money in for the future, right? College is an investment for the future. At conferences, so many things are often suggested: Use your wealth to put into that, to get the connections, to get this, and to get that. And then it's going to pay off later. But what if you don't have that startup money, right?

We have to think differently about our teacher-scholar pipeline and how we are making sure that we're providing resources for people; We need to begin an investment in them because they don't have it and many times students/ people of color already are not only providing for themselves, but they're providing for their families who are often coming from these working-class backgrounds.

Excerpt of Maryland 2023 Moore-Miller Transition Report (Governor, Wes Moore; Lt. Governor, Aruna Miller)

One of the significant themes that emerged from the work of the Education Policy Committee that Dr. Edwards advised was to support students from marginalized communities. Special Education Services is included as one of the beneficiaries of increased funding. Outlined in pages 40 & 41, are the following:

Appendix G: Interview with Professor Dr. Norell Edwards

Provide better services for students with disabilities. Strengthening the pipeline of special education teachers and providing high-quality instruction and services to students with disabilities will enable Maryland to meet the needs of all students and families. Success requires strengthening career pipelines for special educators and increasing state-level support for students with disabilities. The state will need to engage students with disabilities, their families and caregivers, educators, out-of-school time and community-based program providers, the Governor's Office of Children, local education agencies, MSDE, the Maryland Department of Disability (MDOD), and the Special Education Advisory Committee.

Recommended short-term actions:

- Convene stakeholders from around the state to learn what's working and what's not for students with disabilities and their families.

- Strengthen the pipeline of special education teachers by implementing the Blueprint for Maryland Future's Pillar II pay increases.

- Create new state-level standards to hold local education authorities accountable for provisions of appropriate evidence-based services.

Recommended long-term actions:

Develop a plan to increase slots in teacher preparation programs focused on special education.

- Provide incentives for students pursuing degrees in special education.

- Ensure all teacher training programs include some training on how to support students with disabilities.

- Ensure the Service Year Option Program includes a special education track and support other pipeline and internship programs that recruit students to special education-focused internships.

- Create statewide recommended student-teacher ratios based on the diverse needs of students with disabilities.

Measures of Success

The state will need to monitor (1) the increase in the number of people with disabilities who obtain competitive employment; (2) the reduction in disparate discipline rates for students with disabilities; (3) the increase in retention rates of special educators; and (4) reductions in achievement gaps between students with disabilities and general education students.

References

Alegria, M., Vallas, M., Pumariega, A., (2010). Racial and Ethnic Disparities in Pediatric Mental Health. *Child Adolescent Psychiatry Clinics of North America*, 194: 759-774.

Amato PR, Patterson S, Beattie B. Single-Parent Households and Children's Educational Achievement: A State-Level Analysis. *Social Science Research*, 53:191-202.

APA Task Force on Race and Ethnicity Guidelines in Psychology (2019). Race and Ethnicity Guidelines in Psychology: Promoting Responsiveness and Equity. *American Psychological Association (APA)*.

Anderson, C. (2018). A Black History Reader; 101 Questions You Never Thought to Ask. *PowerNomics Corporation of America, Inc.*

Anderson, J. (2020). Harvard Podcast: Racial Differences in Special Education Identification. *Harvard Graduate School of Education*.

Baum, D. (2016, April). Legalize it all. *Harper's Magazine*.

Battery, Dan & Leyva, Luis & Williams, Immanuel & Belizario, Victoria & Grego, Rachel & Shah, Roshini. (2018). Racial (Mis)Match in Middle School Mathematics Classrooms: Relational Interactions as a Racialized Mechanism. *Harvard Educational Review*. 88. 455-482.

Benson, P. L., Roehlkepartain, E. C., & Rude, S. P. (2003). Benson, P. L., Roehlkepartain, E. C., & Rude, S. P. (2003). Spiritual development in childhood and adolescence: Toward a field of inquiry. *Applied Developmental Science,* 7(3), 205–213. https://doi.org/10.1207/S1532480XADS0703_12

Black, H. G. (1947). *The Bible in American Schools. Christian Education, 30(4),* 314–322. http://www.jstor.org/stable/41175248

Blackwell, Angela Glover (2017). The Curb-Cut Effect. *Stanford Social Innovation Review,* Winter 2017.

Board of Governors of the Federal Reserve System (2019). *Survey of Consumer Finances.*

Brazelton, T. B. (2006). Touchpoints: The Essential Reference. *Da Capo Press.*

Breen, Patrick (2020). *Nat Turner's Revolt (1831). Encyclopedia Virginia.*

Brockett, R.G, & Hiemstra, R. (1991). Self-direction in Adult Learning: Perspectives on Theory, Research and Practice (1st ed.). *Routledge.* https://doi.org/10.4324/9780429457319

Brown-Chidsey, R., & Steege, M. W. (2010). Response to Intervention: Principles and Strategies for Effective Practice (2nd ed.). *Guilford Press.*

Brown, H. C., & H, B. M. (2019). Preparing Trauma-Sensitive Teachers: Strategies for Teacher Educators. *Teacher Educators' Journal* 12th ed., pg. 129–152.

Cai, W., Duberg, K., Padmanabhan, A., Rehert, R., Bradley, T., Carrion, V., & Menon, V. (2019). Hyperdirect insula-basal-ganglia pathway and adult-like maturity of global brain responses predict inhibitory control in children. *Nature Communications,* 10(1), 4798. https://doi.org/10.1038/s41467-019-12756-8

Carmody, Steve (2024). It's been 10 years since the start of a devastating water crisis in Flint, Mich. *National Public Radio.*

References

Cavanagh, C., Paruk, J., & Grisso, T. (2022). The developmental reform in juvenile justice: Its progress and vulnerability. *Psychology, Public Policy, and Law*, 28(2), 151–166.

Cecelski, D.S. (2016). Along Freedom Road: Hyde County, North Carolina, and the Fate of Black Schools in the South. *University of North Carolina Press.*

Center for Disease Control (2019). National Center on Birth Defects and Developmental Disabilities.

Chen, C., Li, Z., Liu, X., Pan, Y., & Wu, T. (2022). Cognitive Control Deficits in Children With Subthreshold Attention-Deficit/Hyperactivity Disorder. *Frontiers in Human Neuroscience*, 16. https://doi.org/10.3389/fnhum.2022.835544

Chin, M. J., Quinn, D. M., Dhaliwal, T. K., & Lovison, V. S. (2020). Bias in the Air: A Nationwide Exploration of Teachers' Implicit Racial Attitudes, Aggregate Bias, and Student Outcomes. *Educational Researcher*, 49(8), 566–578.

Coates, T. (2018). We Were Eight Years in Power: An American Tragedy. *One World.*

Connelly, Eileen (2008). Overlooked No More: Brad Lomax, a Bridge Between Civil Rights Movements. *The New York Times.*

Constantino, J. N., Abbacchi, A. M., Saulnier, C., Klaiman, C., Mandell, D. S., Zhang, Y., Hawks, Z., Bates, J., Klin, A., Shattuck, P., Molholm, S., Fitzgerald, R., Roux, A., Lowe, J. K., & Geschwind, D. H. (2020). *Timing of the Diagnosis of Autism in African American Children. Pediatrics*, 146(3), e20193629.

Counts, J., Katsiyannis, A. & Whitford, K. (2018). Culturally and Linguistically Diverse Learners in Special Education: English Learners. *NASSP Bulletin* 102 (1): 5–21.

Craft, S. (2023). The Death Penalty in Decline. *Equal Justice USA*.

Cross, T. L., Benjamin, M. P., & Isaacs, M. R. (1989). Towards a culturally competent system of care. CASSP Technical Assistance Center, Georgetown University Child Development Center. What Are Adverse Childhood Experiences (ACES)? *Resilient Child Fund*.

Davis, T., Harrison, L. (2013). Advancing Social Justice: Tools, Pedagogies, and Strategies to Transform Your Campus. *Jossey-Bass*.

Degner, J. (2017). Culturally Responsive Teaching and the UDL Connection. BCSC/CAST, 24–25. *Learningdesigned.org*.

Department of Education Open Data Platform. Data Profiles. *Data.ed.gov*.

Department of Education Sends Letter to State Directors of Special Education About Highly Mobile Children (2022). *Individuals with Disabilities Education Act*.

Derman-Sparks, L., & Philips, C. B. (1997). Teaching/Learning Anti-Racism: A Developmental Approach. *Teachers College Press*.

Division of Special Education/Early Intervention Services (2013). Role of the School Psychologist in the Identification of Emotional Disability Guidance and Technical Assistance for School Psychologists In Assessment, Identification, Service Provision, and Progress Monitoring of Students with Emotional Disability. *Maryland State Department of Education*.

Duncan, A. (2010). Free Appropriate Public Education Under Section 504 of The Rehabilitation Act (1973).

Duncan, A. & Lhamon, C. (2014). Civil Rights Data Collection, Data Snapshot: School Discipline. Department of EducationDunson, W. E. (2013). School Success for Kids with Dyslexia & Other Reading Difficulties. *Prufrock Press*.

References

Dryden, Jum (2020). African American children with autism experience long delays in diagnosis. *Washington University School of Medicine in St. Louis.*

Edwards, F., Lee, H., & Esposito, M. (2019). Risk of Being Killed by Police Use of Force in the United States by Age, Race–Ethnicity, and Sex. *Proceedings of the National Academy of Sciences*, 116(34), 16793–16798.

Feinberg, E., Silverstein, M., Donahue, S., & Bliss, R. (2011). The impact of race on participation in part C early intervention services. *Journal of Developmental and Behavioral Pediatric*, 32(4), 284–291. https://doi.org/10.1097/DBP.0b013e3182142fbd.

Fletcher-Janzen, E., Strickland, T. L., & Reynolds, C. R. (2000). Handbook of Cross-Cultural Neuropsychology. *Kluwer Academic/Plenum Publishers.*

Freire, P. (1972). Pedagogy of the Oppressed: Translated. by Myra Bergman Ramos. *Herder and Herder.*

Fujii, D. (2017). Conducting a Culturally Informed Neuropsychological Evaluation. *American Psychological Association.*

Gabarino, J. (2000). Lost Boys: Why Our Sons Turn Violent and How We Can Save Them. *Anchor*

Gao, N., & Hayes, J. (2021). The Digital Divide in Education. *Public Policy Institute of California.*

Gary, F. A. (2005). Stigma: Barrier to Mental Health Care Among Ethnic Minorities. *Mental Health Nursing*, 26(10), 979–999.

Gay, G. (2018). Culturally Responsive Teaching: Theory, Research, and Practice. *Teachers College Press.*

Gill, C. S., Barrio Minton, C. A., & Myers, J. E. (2010). Spirituality and religiosity: Factors affecting wellness among low-income, rural women. *Journal of Counseling & Development*, 88(3), 293–302.

Gillespie, K. M., Kemps, E., White, M. J., & Bartlett, S. E. (2023). The impact of free sugar on human health—a narrative review. *Nutrients*, 15(4), 889. https://doi.org/10.3390/nu15040889.

Goldthree, R. (2016). Prefiguring the African American "Postcolony": Black Independent Schools and the Quest for Liberation. *African American Intellectual History Society*.

Gondré-Lewis, M.C., Abijo, T. & Gondré-Lewis, T.A (2023). The Opioid Epidemic: a Crisis Disproportionately Impacting Black Americans and Urban Communities. *Journal Racial and Ethnic Health Disparities*, 10, 2039–2053. https://doi.org/10.1007/s40615-022-01384-6.

Gordon, N. (2017, September 20). Race, poverty, and interpreting overrepresentation in special education. *Brookings Institute*.

Gottfried, M. A. (2019). Chronic Absenteeism in the Classroom Context: Effects on Achievement. *Urban Education*, 54(1), 3–34. https://doi.org/10.1177/0042085915618709.

Gregory, A., & Weinstein, R. S. (2008). The discipline gap and African Americans: defiance or cooperation in the high school classroom. Journal of School Psychology, 46(4), 455–475. https://doi.org/10.1016/j.jsp.2007.09.001.

Gromball, J., et. al (2014). Hyperactivity, concentration difficulties and impulsiveness improve during seven weeks' treatment with valerian root and lemon balm extracts in primary school children. *Phytomedicine*, 21 (8–9).

References

Hamaji, K., & Terenzi, K. (2021). Arrested Learning - A survey of youth experiences of police and security at school Arrested Learning. *Center for Popular Democracy.*

Harry, B., & Klingner, J. K. (2014). Why Are So Many Minority Students in Special Education?: Understanding Race & Disability In Schools. *Teachers College Press.*

Hoffman, K. M., Trawalter, S., Axt, J. R., & Oliver, M. N. (2016). Racial Bias in Pain Assessment and Treatment Recommendations, and False Beliefs about Biological Differences between Blacks and Whites. *Proceedings of the National Academy of Sciences*, 113(16), 4296–4301.

Honsinger, C. & Brown, M. H. (2019). Preparing trauma-sensitive teachers: Strategies for teacher educators. *Teacher Educators' Journal*, 12, 129-15.

hooks, b. (1984). Feminist Theory: from margin to center. *Routledge, Taylor & Francis Group.*

hooks, b. (1989). Talking Back- Thinking Feminist, Thinking Black. *Routledge, Taylor & Francis Group.*

hooks, b. (1990). Yearning: Race, Gender, and Cultural Politics. *Routledge, Taylor & Francis Group.*

House & Toporek (2022). American Counseling Association Advocacy Competencies. *ACA Advocacy Competencies.*

Illinois ACEs Response Collaborative. (n.d.). Education Brief: Aces for Educators and Stakeholders. *Health & Medicine Policy Research Group.*

Inside Institute of Education Science (n.d.). IES Announces a New Research and Development Center for Self-Directed Learning Skills in Online College Courses. *Ies.ed.gov.*

Institute of Education Sciences (2021). NCER's Investments in Education Research Networks to Accelerate Pandemic Recovery Network Lead Spotlight: Dr. Rebecca Griffiths. *LEARN Network.*

Institute of Education Sciences (2022). School Pulse Panel 2021–22 and 2022–23. *National Center for Education Statistics.*

Inquiry Commissions of Inquiry (2021) International Commission of Inquiry on Systemic Racist Police Violence Against People of African Descent in the United States. *Nathaniel Pickett II Hearing.*

International Commission of Inquiry (2021). Report of the International Commission of Inquiry on Systemic Racist Police Violence against People of African Descent in the United States.

James & Jackson (2021). Addressing Implicit Bias among Psychologists, Physicians, and School Staff. *American Psychological Association.*

Jackson K. & Jackson M. (2021), P.A.R.E.N.T.S. Life Skills, Literacy, & Leadership 2nd Edition. *Shamen Resh Institute.*

John Hopkins School of Education. (2017). May 2017 Restorative Practices in Schools Prepared for the Open Society Institute. *Attendance Works.*

Jordan, P. (2019). Tapping Federal Dollars to Reduce Chronic Absenteeism. *FutureEd.*

Kenney, E. L., Long, M. W., Cradock, A. L., & Gortmaker, S. L. (2015). Prevalence of Inadequate Hydration Among US Children and Disparities by Gender and Race/Ethnicity: National Health and Nutrition Examination Survey, 2009-2012. *American Journal of Public*

Health, 105(8), e113–e118. https://doi.org/10.2105/AJPH.2015.302572.

Kunjufu, J. (1985). Countering the Conspiracy to Destroy Black Boys; Vol. I. *African American Images*.

Lanark County County Justice. (n.d.). What are Restorative Practices?

Lange, R.T. (2011). Full Scale IQ. In: Kreutzer, J.S., DeLuca, J., Caplan, B. (eds) Encyclopedia of Clinical Neuropsychology. *Springer*. https://doi.org/10.1007/978-0-387-79948-3_1549.

LearningforJustice.org (2022). Food Desert Statistics. *Teaching Tolerance*.

Lehr, J., McComas, W. F., & Chakroborti, S. (2006). Cultural Comparisons and Implications for Students With Ebd: A Decade Of Understanding. *International Journal of Special Education*, 25 (9).

Losen, D. J., & Orfield, G. (2002). Racial Inequality in Special Education. *ResearchGate*.

Lustig, R. H. (2010). Fructose: metabolic, hedonic, and societal parallels with ethanol. *Journal of the American Dietetic Association,* 110(9), 1307-1321.

Lynn, Samara (2020, January 19). Controversial Group ADOS Divides Black Americans in Fight for Economic Equality. *ABC News*.

MacPherson, K. (2008). Sugar can be addictive, Princeton scientist says. *Princeton University*.

Mandell, D. S., Wiggins, L. D., Carpenter, L. A., Daniels, J., DiGuiseppi, C., Durkin, M. S., Giarelli, E., Morrier, M. J., Nicholas, J. S., Pinto-Martin, J. A., Shattuck, P. T., Thomas, K. C., Yeargin-Allsopp, M., & Kirby, R. S. (2009). Racial/ethnic disparities in the identification of children with autism spectrum disorders. *American Journal of*

Public Health, 99(3), 493-498. https://doi.org/10.2105/AJPH.2007.131243

Marengo, Katherine & Eske, Jamie (2019). What are the health benefits of mineral water? *Medical News Today.*

Morgan, Hani. (2020). "Misunderstood and Mistreated: Students of Color in Special Education." *Voices of Reform: Educational Research to Inform and Reform* 3 (2): 71–81. https://doi.org/10.32623/3.10005.

Pinto-Martin, J. A., Shattuck, P. T., Thomas, K. C., Yeargin-Allsopp, M., & Kirby, R. S. (2009). Racial/Ethnic Disparities in the Identification of Children With Autism Spectrum Disorders. *American Journal of Public Health,* 99(3), 493–498.

Marquad, R. (1985). The rise and fall of the Bible in US classrooms. As the outcry grows to 'get religion back into the classroom,' the Monitor looks at the historic role of the Bible in American public schools. *Christian Science Monitor.*

McCord, J., & Tremblay, R. E. (1992). Preventing Antisocial Behavior: Interventions from Birth Through Adolescence. *The Guilford Press,* 6(1), 1–20.

McGuinness, D. (1999). Why Our Children Can't Read and What We Can Do About It: A Scientific Revolution in Reading. *Simon & Schuster.*

Mcnair, T., Bensimon, E., Malcom-Piqueux, L. E., (2020). From Equity Talk to Equity Walk: Expanding Practitioner Knowledge for Racial Justice in Higher Education. *Association Of American Colleges and Universities, & Jossey-Bass Inc.*

Moats, L. C. (2015). Teaching Adolescents to Read: It is Not Too Late. *Edweek,* 1–12.

References

Morgan, H. (2020). Misunderstood and Mistreated: Students of Color in Special Education. *Voices of Reform*, 3(2), 71–81.

Morgan, P. L. (2021). Unmeasured Confounding and Racial or Ethnic Disparities in Disability Identification. *Educational Evaluation and Policy Analysis*, 43(2), 351-361. https://doi.org/10.3102/0162373721991575.

Morgan, P. L., Staff, J., Hillemeier, M. M., Farkas, G., & Maczuga, S. (2013). Racial and ethnic disparities in ADHD diagnosis from kindergarten to eighth grade. *Pediatrics*, 132(1), 85–93. https://doi.org/10.1542/peds.2012-2390.

My Brother's Keeper Alliance (2021). *Obama Foundation.*

Naftali, T. (2019). Ronald Reagan's Long-Hidden Racist Conversation With Richard Nixon In newly unearthed audio, the then–California governor disparaged African delegates to the United Nations. *The Atlantic.*

National Center for Education and Statistics (2020). Data Point- Race and Ethnicity of Public School Teachers and Their Students. *Department of Education, Institute of Education Sciences.*

National Center for Education Statistics. (2021). Digest of Education Statistics. Department of Education, *Institute of Education Sciences.*

National Center for Education Statistics. (2023). Students With Disabilities. Condition of Education. Department of Education, *Institute of Education Sciences.*

National Center for Learning Disabilities (2020). Significant Disproportionality in Special Education: Trends Among Black Students. *Indian Council of Administrators of Special. Education.*

National Research Council. 2002. Minority Students in Special and Gifted Education. *The National Academies Press.* https://doi.org/10.17226/10128.

National Conference of Black Lawyers United States. (n.d.). NCBL.

Obasogie, O. (2021). Excited Delirium and police use of force. *Virginia Law,* 107 (8).

Office of The Surgeon General, Center For Mental Health Services, U. S. & National Institute Of Mental Health, U. S. (1999). Mental health: a report of the Surgeon General. *United States Public Health Service.*

Partners for Each and Every Child. (2017). A District Guide to ESSA and the Importance of Stakeholder Engagement Participation, Preparation & What Comes Next. *Opportunity Institute,* 1-20.

Patel, A. I., & Hampton, K. E. (2011). Encouraging consumption of water in school and child care settings: access, challenges, and strategies for improvement. *American Journal of Public Health,* 101(8), 1370–1379. https://doi.org/10.2105/AJPH.2011.300142.

Patrick, K., Onyeka-Crawford, A., & Duchesneau, N. "...And they cared": How To Create Better, Safer Learning Environment for Girls of Color. *The Education Trust,* 1–26.

Perception Institute. (2019). Perception Institute. https://perception.org/.

Peters, S. J., Gentry, M., Whiting, G. W., & McBee, M. T. (2019). Who Gets Served in Gifted Education? Demographic Representation and a Call for Action. *Gifted Child Quarterly,* 63(4), 273–287.

Peterson, Karen (2023). Are you drinking water all wrong? Here's what you need to know about hydrating. Salted? Alkaline? Here's what you actually need to hydrate. *National Geographic.*

Posner, L. (2021). I was a well-meaning White teacher, But my Harsh Discipline Harmed Black Kids. *Washington Post.*

Quattrini, S., Pampaloni, B., & Brandi, M. L. (2016). Natural mineral waters: chemical characteristics and health effects. Clinical cases in mineral and bone metabolism. *Journal of the Italian Society of Osteoporosis, Mineral Metabolism, and Skeletal Diseases,* 13(3), 173–180.

Quinn, M. M., Rutherford, R. B., Leone, P. E., Osher, D. M., & Poirier, J. M. (2005). Youth with Disabilities in Juvenile Corrections: A National Survey. *Exceptional Children,* 71(3), 339–345.

United States Government Accountability Office (2018). K-12 EDUCATION Discipline Disparities for Black Students, Boys, and Students with Disabilities. *Report to Congressional Requesters.*

United States Government Accountability Office (2019). Special education: Idea dispute resolution activity in selected states varied based on school districts' characteristics.

Reimagining the Role of Technology in Education: 2017 National Education Technology Plan Update (2017). *U.S. Department of Education.*

Report to Congressional Requesters (2018). K-12 EDUCATION Discipline Disparities for Black Students, Boys, and Students with Disabilities. *United States Government Accountability Office.*

Rickford, R. (2017). The Pragmatic Utopia: An Author's Response. *African American Intellectual History Society.*

Rios V. & Galicia M. (2013). Smoking guns or smoke & mirrors?: Schools and the policing of Latino boys. *Association of Mexican American Educators Journal,* 2013.

Ripat, J., & Woodgate, R. (2011). The intersection of culture, disability and assistive technology. Disability and rehabilitation. *Assistive Technology,* 6(2), 87–96. https://doi.org/10.3109/17483107.2010.507859.

Rowe, S. W. (2020) Healing Racial Trauma: The Road to Resilience. *IVP, Intervarsity Press.*

Rubenstein, M. (2022). H.B. 23 Department of Legislative Services – Maryland. *Maryland General Assembly.*

Rutter, V. B. (2002). Celebrating Girls. *Inner Ocean Publishing.*

Sabin, J., Nosek, B., Greenwald, A., & Rivara, F. (2009). Physicians' Implicit and Explicit Attitudes About Race by MD Race, Ethnicity, and Gender. *Journal of Health Care for the Poor and Underserved,* 20(3), 896–913.

Sen, Amartya (1983). Poverty: Identification and Aggregation, Poverty and Famines: An Essay on Entitlement and Deprivation. *Oxford Academic.* https://doi.org/10.1093/0198284632.003.0003.

Shankman, S. A., Lewinsohn, P. M., Klein, D. N., Small, J. W., Seeley, J. R., & Altman, S. E. (2009). Subthreshold conditions as precursors for full syndrome disorders: A 15-year longitudinal study of multiple diagnostic classes. *Journal of Child Psychology and Psychiatry,* 50(12), 1485-1494. https://doi.org/10.1111/j.1469-7610.2009.02117.x.

Singer, T., & Lamm, C. (2009). The Social Neuroscience of Empathy. *Annals of the New York Academy of Sciences,* 1156(1), 81–96.

Skiba, R., Artiles, A. J., Kozleski, E. B., Losen, D., & Harry, B. (2016). Risks and consequences of over-simplifying educational inequities: A response to Morgan et al. (2015). *Educational Researcher,* 45, 221-225.

Slavin, R. E. (2021). Educational Psychology: Theory and Practice (12th ed.). *Pearson.*

Smedley, B. D., Stith, A. Y., & Nelson, A. R. (2003). Unequal Treatment: Confronting Racial and Ethnic Disparities in Health Care. *The National Academies Press.*

South Carolina. State Agricultural Society (1848). The negro law of South Carolina. O'Neall, J. B., comp Columbia, Printed by J.G. Bowman. https://www.loc.gov/item/10034474/.

Spiegelman, M. (2020). Race and Ethnicity of Public School Teachers and Their Students. *National Center for Education Statistics.*

Spiritual Development in Childhood and Adolescence: Toward a Field of Inquiry. *Applied Developmental Science,* 7(3), 205–213. https://doi.org/10.1207/s1532480xads0703_12.

Stiefel, L., Shiferaw, M., Schwartz, A. E., & Gottfried, M. (2018). Who Feels Included in School? Examining Feelings of Inclusion Among Students With Disabilities. *Educational Researcher,* 47(2), 105-120. https://doi.org/10.3102/0013189X17738761.

Stringer, A.Y. (2011). Neuropsychology. In: Kreutzer, J.S., DeLuca, J., Caplan, B. (eds) *Encyclopedia of Clinical Neuropsychology.* Springer. https://doi.org/10.1007/978-0-387-79948-3_671.

Task Force on Achieving Academic Equity and Excellence for Black Boys (2021). Transforming the Culture of Maryland's Schools for Black Boys; A Resource Guide for Educators. *Maryland Public Schools.*

The Conversation (2019). What Daniel Patrick Moynihan Actually Thought About Race. *The Atlantic.*

The Education Trust (2022). Recommendations for Congress- Child Nutrition Reauthorization. *EdTrust.org.*

Thompson, C. (2021). Fatal Police Shootings of Unarmed Black People Reveal Troubling Patterns. *National Public Radio.*

Tisdell, E. (2001). Spirituality in adult and higher education. *Eric Digests.*

Tucker, B., & Mitchell-Kernan, C. (1995). The Decline in Marriage Among African Americans: Causes, Consequences, and Policy Implications. *Russell Sage Foundation.*

Trent, M., Dooley, D. G., & Dougé, J. (2019). The Impact of Racism on Child and Adolescent Health. *Pediatrics,* 144(2), e20191765. *American Academy of Pediatrics.*

Tresco K.E., Lefler E.K., & Power, T.J. (2010). Psychosocial Interventions to Improve the School Performance of Students with Attention-Deficit/Hyperactivity Disorder. *Mind Brain,* 1(2):69-74.

United States Congress Address (1986). Anti-Drug Abuse Act of 1986. National Criminal Justice Reference Service. *Office of Justice Programs.*

United States Congress Address (1984). Comprehensive Crime Control Act of 1984. *Office of Justice Programs.*

United States Department of Agriculture (2020). Dietary Guidelines for Americans 2020-2025. *Office of Disease Prevention and Promotion.*

United States Department of Education (2019) Guide to the Individualized Education Program. *Office of Special Education and Rehabilitative Services.*

Valencia, R. R. (2010). Dismantling Contemporary Deficit Thinking: Educational Thought and Practice. *Routledge.*

Washington, Booker T. (1901). Up From Slavery: An Autobiography. *Rare Book Collection, University of North Carolina at Chapel Hill.*

References

Wisconsin Department of Health Services (2024). Resilient Wisconsin: Adverse Childhood Experiences. What are adverse childhood experiences? *State of Wisconsin.*

University of Washington (2022). What is the Difference Between an IEP and a 504 Plan? https://www.washington.edu/doit/what-difference-between-iep-and-504-plan

Weathers, Saundra (2020). Justice for All: Racial Disparities for Bay Area Black Children? *Spectrum Bay News 9.*

Weinfeld, R. & Neu, T. W. (2007). Helping Boys Succeed in School: A Practical Guide for Parents and Teachers. *Prufrock Press.*

William, F. A, Charles, P. W., & Garrison, L. M. (1867). Slave songs of the United States. *New York, A. Simpson & Co.*

Wright, J. L., Davis, W. S., Joseph, M. M., Ellison, A. M., Heard-Garris, N. J., Johnson, T. L., & the AAP Board Committee on Equity (2022). Eliminating Race-Based Medicine. *American Academy of Pediatrics.*

Wright, P.D. & Wright, P. (2021). The History of Special Education Law in the United States. *Wrights Law.*

W3C Working Group (2019). Making Content Usable for People with Cognitive and Learning Disabilities. *World Wide Web Consortium (W3C).*

Zakrzewski, V. (2013). The case for discussing spirituality in schools. *Greater Good Magazine.*

Zippia (2021). Special Education Teacher Demographics and Statistics https://www.zippia.com/special-education-teacher-jobs/demographics/

About the Author

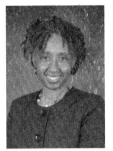

Marcy Rachamim Jackson, M.A. is a compassionate education consultant with 30 years of experience across higher education, special education advocacy, and workforce education.

With practice and research interests in equity, disability, education, leadership, and parenting, she is the Founding Coordinator of the nonprofit initiative SEE US: Special Education Excellence for Underserved Students, improving the special education experience for Black students with special needs.

Mrs. Jackson is a special education equity justice champion, aware of the disability education ecosystem and is highly sensitive to the disparities that exist for Black students in particular, with special needs.

Alongside her husband, she is a special needs parent and the coauthor of *P.A.R.E.N.T.S. Life Skills, Literacy, and Leadership Framework for Social Change*©, a prison and reentry program for reparenting. Mrs. Jackson provides education consulting through Olivez Education Grove, LLC. She resides in Maryland, where she delights in quality faith and family time.

Made in the USA
Middletown, DE
25 May 2025